The Public Health Crisis Survival Guide

LEADERSHIP AND MANAGEMENT
IN TRYING TIMES

JOSHUA M. SHARFSTEIN

*Professor of the Practice, Department of Health Policy
    and Management*
*Vice Dean for Public Health Practice and Community
    Engagement*
Johns Hopkins Bloomberg School of Public Health

OXFORD
UNIVERSITY PRESS

OXFORD
UNIVERSITY PRESS

Oxford University Press is a department of the University of Oxford. It furthers
the University's objective of excellence in research, scholarship, and education
by publishing worldwide. Oxford is a registered trade mark of Oxford University
Press in the UK and certain other countries.

Published in the United States of America by Oxford University Press
198 Madison Avenue, New York, NY 10016, United States of America.

Library of Congress Cataloging-in-Publication Data
Names: Sharfstein, Joshua M., author.
Title: The public health crisis survival guide: leadership and management
in trying times / Joshua M. Sharfstein.
Description: Oxford; New York: Oxford University Press, [2018] |
Includes bibliographical references and index.
Identifiers: LCCN 2017049326 | ISBN 9780190697211 (pbk.: alk. paper)
Subjects: | MESH: Public Health Administration—methods |
Public Health Administration—trends | Government Agencies—organization & administration |
Health Policy | Safety Management | United States Classification:
LCC RA971 | NLM WA 540 AA1 | DDC 362.1068—dc23
LC record available at https://lccn.loc.gov/2017049326

9 8 7 6 5 4 3 2

Printed by Webcom, Inc., Canada

The Public Health Crisis Survival Guide

For Yngvild

CONTENTS

On my first day as a faculty member of the School of Public Health, my department chair Dr. Ellen MacKenzie asked me to develop a course for graduate students.

"Whatever you'd like," she said.

I quickly drafted a syllabus for a class to be titled Politics and Public Health. I thought to myself: Why not? During 15 years working in the public sector, I experienced political pressures of all kinds. I had served as professional staff for a member of Congress, as health commissioner for two mayors, as health secretary for a governor, and as acting commissioner and principal deputy commissioner at the U.S. Food and Drug Administration.

"This will be easy," I imagined as I submitted my syllabus for approval to the school's Committee on Academic Standards.

Rejected. The Committee's terse explanation to me: "There already is a course on politics and public health."

I tried again. This time, my proposed course was to be called Solving Problems in Public Health. I based the syllabus on several thorny decisions that confronted me in the public sector.

No thanks, said the Committee. Problem Solving in Public Health is already one of our most popular courses.

Public health policy? Taken. Public health advocacy? Two courses already. Eventually, I paused and returned, defeated, to my department chair.

Instead of developing a course that you believe would be easy to teach, Dr. MacKenzie suggested, how about creating one that you wish you had taken? Surely, she said, you didn't know everything before working in public health?

And then it hit me.

Crisis.

How unprepared I had been for the multiple crises that came to dominate so much of my time in various positions. One of our agency programs overspends the budget by millions, leading to a frantic search for more funding? Crisis. A different program underspends the budget by millions, with those who would have benefitted from the foregone funds marching on the State House? Crisis.

Auditors finding inadequate oversight of healthcare facilities? A potential Ebola case in a local emergency department? A fatal outbreak at a cosmetic surgery center? Patient-on-patient violence at one of our mental health facilities? Crisis, crisis, crisis, crisis.

I had learned the hard way that what counts as a public health crisis is not easily described nor measured; there is no formula with a cutoff score. A crisis involves the sense that a great deal is at stake. It's that moment when the competence and even the purpose of the agency and its leadership are tested, and reputations hang in the balance. In a crisis, what happens next really matters.

Many graduate courses teach a step-by-step approach to tackling challenges in public health, but life in the field can be anything but rational. My proposed class would take crisis from the background and place it squarely in the foreground.

Crisis not as an interruption to the work of public health but as a major part of the work itself, to be studied and understood.

Crisis not just as a problem to be prevented through diligent public health work but as a fact of life that requires attention now.

Crisis not as a misery to be endured but as an opportunity for unexpected progress.

The Committee on Academic Standards responded: "Do you mean disaster management? That class is already offered in the fourth term."

No, I pleaded. Unlike disaster management, my class would cover more than operational issues. It would cover the history, context, and strategy of crisis—along the way engaging with politics, problem-solving, policy, and advocacy. The goal would be to equip students interested in serving in a variety of health agency management roles with a set of skills and a level of confidence for handling all kinds of existential challenges, from the predictable to the unexpected.

Finally, the Committee said yes—and I've enjoyed immensely teaching the class, now called Crisis and Response in Public Health Policy and Practice. For their written assignments, my students pick crises of the last century, assess what happened, and suggest what might have been done differently—fan fiction for public health.

My involvement with public health crises has extended beyond the classroom. About every week or so, I hear from a local, state, or federal health official wanting to talk through a crisis facing his or her own agency. We discuss rising opioid overdoses, irate city council members, coming fiscal calamities, human resources meltdowns, and critical audit reports. Many of those calling have been former colleagues, now in charge; others have just heard that I'm available to listen and offer ideas to help with thorny challenges.

I very much enjoy supporting great people in the field of public health manage and lead through crises, big or small. I especially appreciate the moment in our conversations when new ideas start to surface and the clouds begin to part. Even over the phone, I can recognize a palpable sense of relief—and of resolve.

The goal of this book is put in writing what I have learned from these experiences—and to continue this quest to assist current and future health officials find success in the most difficult and trying of times.

ACKNOWLEDGMENTS

B ecause this book started with *300.650.01: Crisis and Response in Public Health Policy and Practice*, I owe my first thanks to those who made this course possible. The list includes my former chair of the Department of Health Policy and Management (and current Dean of the Johns Hopkins Bloomberg School of Public Health) Ellen MacKenzie, former Dean Mike Klag, current chair Colleen Barry, and two terrific teaching assistants, Rachel Fabi and Amelie Hecht. I also thank Vicente Navarro for permission to teach the class over two days in Barcelona at our Institute held jointly with the Universidad Pompeo Fabra, and Dr. Carme Borrell, the health commissioner of Barcelona for the participation of her great Department. The course would not be what it is without my fantastic guest lecturers, including FDA historian John Swann (who also provided sources for the FDA chapters), former CDC official Edward Hunter, David Peters and the inspiring Tolbert Nyenswah on Ebola, and biosecurity expert Jennifer Nuzzo. Most of all, I appreciate the energy, intelligence, and acumen of more than 200 students who have taken the class so far.

This is also an appropriate time to thank those who made it possible for me to teach a class or write a book on this topic. This group starts with my first employer after I finished my pediatric training, Congressman Henry A. Waxman, whose strategic sense and judgment in the service of smart health policy is second to none. I learned so much from him and his brilliant staff, including Phil Barnett, Karen Nelson, Phil Schiliro, Karen Lightfoot, Sarah Despres, Brian Cohen, and many others. I thank then-Mayor Martin O'Malley and City Council President (and later Mayor) Sheila Dixon for taking a risk and hiring me as health commissioner for

Baltimore, and for supporting innovative and bold ideas that reduced drug overdoses, violence, and infant mortality, while improving vaccination rates and preparation for school. I am proud to have served as an appointee for President Barack Obama under HHS Secretary Kathleen Sebelius and Deputy Secretary William Corr. At FDA, I met thousands of inspiring federal scientists and learned at the side of a true public health hero, Commissioner Margaret Hamburg.

I thank the other teachers I've had along the way, from David Kessler and Ann Witt at FDA (while I was a medical student), to Sidney Wolfe of Public Citizen, to Georges Benjamin of the American Public Health Association, to William Schultz and Nicole Lurie at HHS, to Thomas Frieden of the New York City Health Department, Centers for Disease Control and Prevention, and now RESOLV. I thank Howard Markel for the opportunity to write for *Milbank Quarterly*. Over the years, Howard Bauchner, editor of the *Journal of the American Medical Association*, has taught me so much about clinical care, research, health policy, ethics, and judgment. I owe a special thanks to Governor Martin O'Malley, who hired me again as Secretary of Maryland's Department of Health and Mental Hygiene and instructed me on multiple occasions that my job was never to stop fighting for measurable improvements in health.

Along the way, I've had the chance to work with some truly gifted political staff and pick up from them how to use every (appropriate) trick in the book to get the right thing to happen. These include Matthew Gallagher, Jeanne Hitchcock, John Griffin, and Stephen Neuman. I learned so much from Ralph Tyler that I still hear his voice in my head, and consult it, during difficult times.

The most inspiring part of any career in public health are the people in our field. There are no singular accomplishments. I owe a great debt to Laura Herrera Scott, Olivia Farrow, Gayle Jordan-Randolph, Chuck Milligan, Rianna Matthews-Brown, Dori Henry, Thomas Kim, Lisa Ellis, Katie Burns, and many others. I thank Patrick Dooley for his incredible commitment to the people of Maryland as the most able chief of staff in the history of the Department of Health and Mental Hygiene. There is no way to describe Michelle Spencer, who served as chief of staff to the Baltimore City Health Department for nine years, and worked with me at the state level (and now at Johns Hopkins), other than as a force of nature. She can balance more projects on the tip of her finger than anyone else on the planet.

A few of my friends read over parts of the manuscript, none so diligently and helpfully as my college roommate Daniel Mufson. I was lucky to have Grace Mandel in my class the first time I taught it. Recognizing her brilliance, I hired her to be this project's research assistant. She kept the project on deadline and on track, and contributed sidebars along the way. The Centers for Disease Control and Prevention now has the good fortune of having her on the team. Special thanks to the other sidebar authors, including Edward Hunter, Nicole Lurie, Governor O'Malley, and Mark Harrington (whose fascinating contribution to the appendix could be the start of a book all its own).

This book would never have happened without the strong support at every step from Chad Zimmerman at Oxford University Press and his entire team, including Chloe Layman. Chad kept encouraging me to write a book for people to read, which I hope I have delivered.

My brother Dan supported me with his words, advice, and example as an award-winning writer. My sister Sarah kept me going with helpful phrases like, "Why can't you write more like Dan?" I'm counting on my parents Steven and Margaret to submit online reviews, just as they have supported me in everything I've attempted my entire life. In writing about the intersection of politics, policy, and common sense, I am channeling the legacy of my grandparents. Luna deserves an extra treat for her help with the book; she never let me sit at the computer for too long without demanding a walk and allowing me some time to reflect. For many years now, my antidote to frustration and despair has been time with Sam and Isak, two amazing young men ready to take on the world.

Yngvild Olsen is more than a partner in crime. Her contributions to my life, my career, and this book are impossible to enumerate. Here's the best I can do: When I asked her by Jamaica Pond in 1997 (in lieu of a formal marriage proposal), "Are you ready for this?", her answer made everything else possible. This book is for her.

CONTRIBUTORS

Mark Harrington

Edward L. Hunter

Nicole Lurie

Grace Mandel

Governor Martin O'Malley

The Public Health Crisis Survival Guide

1 | Introduction

AFTER A RABID RACCOON ATTACKED a woman on a Baltimore street, knocking her to the ground and biting her, the Baltimore City Health Department was unable to provide the needed rabies shots on time. The day was December 12, 2005—my first on the job as Health Commissioner. I stood at my new desk, holding my new phone, hearing the story from a reporter at the local newspaper, *The Baltimore Sun.*

"How often does the Health Department fail to protect city residents?" he asked. "And is this woman now at risk for rabies?"

I took a short breath and told him I would call him back. I then found out that while the Department promised city residents timely access to the rabies vaccine, the supply had been running low for months (Figure 1.1).

The next morning, I woke up to read in *The Baltimore Sun* that the Health Department had been issuing citations to undergraduates at Loyola University for giving sandwiches to individuals experiencing homelessness in downtown Baltimore.[1] The students lacked access to running water on site, which Health Department regulations apparently required for food preparation. The students were incensed. One was quoted as saying, "If we have food, we're going to feed them. If city officials were hungry and cold, I'm sure they wouldn't want someone to have a license to give them something to eat. It's just stupid. That's what it is."

The following day, I learned that two men experiencing homelessness had died on the streets in the frigid weather, raising questions about the

---

[1] Fuller N. Students still feeding homeless; No city license, no Loyola sponsorship, but charity goes on. *The Baltimore Sun.* 13 December 2005: 3B.

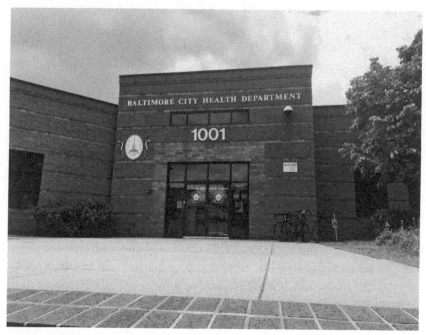

FIGURE 1.1 Baltimore City Health Department
Courtesy Grace Mandel

Department's policy of only opening an emergency shelter at 25 degrees with at least 15 mile-an-hour winds.[2] Reporters asked me to justify the policy.

Two days later—and still during my first week on the job—the Health Department received a warning letter from the U.S. Food and Drug Administration (FDA) threatening to shut down all research at our agency. During an inspection that had occurred six months earlier, the FDA had found major deficiencies with the Department's committee responsible for assuring that research was being conducted ethically. Our Institutional Review Board had been failing to review ongoing projects, failing to hold meetings with requisite attendance, and failing to document informed consent. Yet despite receiving a brutal inspection report, the Health Department had not fixed the problems.

Now the FDA was ready to cancel all 60 or so active research projects, covering, among other areas, the treatment of all the city's patients with active tuberculosis. The infectious disease experts on staff glumly told me that halting the protocols would create a disaster for disease control.

---

[2] Garland G. 2 homeless dead after overnight exposure; third in critical condition after night in sub-freezing weather. *The Baltimore Sun.* 4 December 2005: 1B.

And looming over everything that first week was the impending national transition to Medicare Part D for prescription drug coverage on January 1, 2006—about two weeks away. On that day, about 28,000 of the city's most vulnerable individuals (those "dually eligible" for Medicare and Medicaid) would need to obtain their medications through different insurance, often through different pharmacies. Because many of these medications are essential, such as those that treat diabetes and seizure disorders, even a small amount of trouble figuring out the new system would lead to great harm.[3]

Each of these events distracted me from what I had thought would be my first set of tasks—unpacking my desk, meeting the staff, and getting to know the Health Department. In my mind's eye, I imagined spending my first few months on a listening tour around Baltimore before deciding on a set of strategic priorities.

Instead, my life had become crisis, crisis, crisis.

It did not take me long to realize that my expectations had been backwards. I was not going to have the time and space to pick and choose each of the activities I would work on.

Rather, my activities would be picking me.

Firefighters fight fires. Police race to crime scenes, sirens blaring. Health officials respond to public health crises. Whether health leaders are successful in their positions often depends on how well they can handle a crisis. A solid response generates greater credibility and authority that helps support everything else a health agency does. A bungled response can lead to resignation or dismissal.

This reality comes as a shock to many people who go straight from graduate school or medical practice to the public sector. Many courses in public health schools provide instruction on how to assess problems carefully before designing and weighing options for response. These courses are important, because public health officials must be familiar with evidence on what works, select targets for intervention, and implement projects with competence and diligence.

In a crisis, however, there's often little time to make decisions. What's needed is an ability to manage and communicate in a chaotic environment. Health officials must stand their ground as emotions run high, communities become engaged, politicians lean in, and journalists circle.

In popular imagination, leaders intuitively rise to the challenge of a crisis: Either you have what it takes or you do not. In fact, preparation

---

[3] Salganik MW. City to aid Medicare launch; Health agency to monitor seniors' needs as drug plans shift. *The Baltimore Sun*. 21 December 2005.

is invaluable, and critical skills can be learned and practiced. Students and health officials alike can prepare not only to avoid catastrophe during crises but to set in motion new strategies for health improvement.

Many have heard the saying, often attributed to Chicago Mayor Rahm Emanuel (but apparently more accurately cited to Winston Churchill), "Never let a good crisis go to waste." This is a somewhat blunt way of putting a key point: Crises do create opportunities, and there are responsible ways to seize the moment.

Crises may be born of tragedy, difficult to manage, and exhausting. But they also can lead to important public health progress.

Defining Crisis

The *Oxford English Dictionary* provides three definitions of crisis:

- "a time of intense difficulty or danger,"
- "a time when a difficult or important decision must be made," and
- "the turning point of a disease when an important change takes place, indicating either recovery or death."[4]

All three definitions are useful, but the third may be the most apt. The concept of a "turning point of a disease" derives from clinical medicine, originally describing patients suffering from overwhelming infection. Yet it is relevant to health officials too, because that's what it can feel like to manage through a crisis: Either the agency and its leader will survive—or not.

There is a robust field of study in crisis management, and numerous experts in this field have developed their own definitions of crisis. In 1969, Charles Hermann defined a crisis by three attributes: a threat, a short decision time, and surprise.[5] More recently, Arjen Boin and his colleagues, in their terrific 2005 book, *The Politics of Crisis Management*, described crisis as "a serious threat to the basic structures or the fundamental values and norms of a system, which under time pressure and highly uncertain circumstances necessitates making vital decisions."[6] And Dominic Elliott

---

[4] Wait M, Dictionaries O. *Paperback Oxford English Dictionary.* 7th ed. Oxford: Oxford University Press.
[5] Hermann CF. *Crisis in Foreign Policy: A Simulation Analysis.* Center of International Studies: Princeton University, 1969.
[6] Boin A, Hart P, Stern EJ, Sundelius B. *The Politics of Crisis Management: Public Leadership Under Pressure.* Cambridge, UK: Cambridge University Press, 2005: 2.

and Elliott Smith have noted that "[a] defining characteristic of crisis lies in its symbolism."[7] Their point is that the sense of crisis is elevated when the circumstances raise fundamental questions about whether an agency can meet its core responsibilities.

It is worth noting that none of these definitions treat "crisis" as interchangeable with words like "problem," "disaster," or "challenge." Here's why: A crisis reflects a lot more than the facts of the situation. Certainly, major events such as influenza pandemics will count as crises by any definition. But at the heart of a crisis is a perception of vulnerability, a whiff of panic, a recognition that there's more at stake for an agency and its leader than meets the eye. There's no "homeland security" color code or statistical formula that informs health officials when an issue has reached crisis stage.

In fact, a "crisis" for a health agency need not even be related to a genuine health problem. A critical audit alleging mismanagement, for example, can create a crisis for an official every bit as existential as an outbreak of infectious disease. As one study observed, "A routine incident can trigger a crisis when media and elected leaders frame the incident as an indication of inherent flaws."[8] Failure to take such a situation seriously may be the last mistake a health official makes.

In the business literature, experts have recognized and categorized a broad range of crises. One private-sector list of crisis types includes 10 categories: natural disasters, technical-error accidents, technical-error product harm, human-error accidents, human-error product harm, and workplace violence—as well as rumors, organizational misdeeds, malevolence (such as product tampering), and a category called "challenges," defined as "when the organization is confronted by discontented stakeholders with claims that it is operating in an inappropriate manner."[9]

There's no equivalent list of crisis types for the public sector. But if one did exist, additional categories would have to include budget woes, conflict with other agencies, regulatory inattentiveness, regulatory overzealousness, unpredictable political events, unexpected audit reports, and all of the above triggered by investigative reporting. And that's just the beginning. The responsibilities of health agencies are so vast that the potential

---

[7] Smith D, Elliott D. Exploring the barriers to learning from crisis: Organizational learning and crisis. *Management Learning.* 2007; 38(5): 519–538.

[8] Boin A, Hart P, Stern EJ, Sundelius B. *The Politics of Crisis Management: Public Leadership Under Pressure.* Cambridge, UK: Cambridge University Press, 2005: 3.

[9] Coombs WT. *Ongoing Crisis Communication: Planning, Managing and Responding.* 3rd ed. Los Angeles: SAGE, 2012: 73.

paths to crisis are impossible to enumerate. In fact, it's likely that every health official will have the pleasure of discovering some new ones.

The History of Crisis

Despite the vast number of potential crises in the universe of public health, not everything is new under the sun. A starting point for preparing for crises is appreciating basic themes that have emerged in history. William Faulkner famously wrote, "The past is never dead. It's not even past."[10] These words resonate in public health, where iconic crises shadow subsequent events, even years and decades later.

Some famous crises led to tremendous public health victories. In 1937, after a young agency responded vigorously to an outbreak of deaths caused by a product known as the Elixir Sulfanilamide, the nation focused its attention on establishing a strong food and drug law. The Food, Drug, and Cosmetic Act of 1938 transformed oversight of food and drugs and launched the U.S. Food and Drug Administration into decades of protecting the American people from a broad range of hazards.

Other iconic crises did not have happy endings. In 1976, for example, the Centers for Disease Control and Prevention (CDC) mobilized the nation for a "swine flu" pandemic forecasted to threaten hundreds of thousands or millions of lives. In a key mistake, the government committed to immunizing the entire US population well before such a decision was necessary. Officials also failed to address key logistical challenges, such as how to distribute the vaccine and how to address potential liability on the part of vaccine manufacturers. Compounding these errors, then-President Gerald Ford continued to press forward even after data emerged that the new virus would not become the threat that had been feared. After a few months of controversy, and with just a small fraction of the nation immunized, the CDC halted the program early to investigate severe adverse effects from the vaccine.

Did the nation learn the lessons of the swine flu fiasco? In 2002, during the run-up to the Iraq War, the office of Vice President Dick Cheney spread the word that terrorists in Iraq might have access to stocks of the deadly smallpox virus. As a precaution against a devastating pandemic, the vice president recommended vaccination for the entire US population.[11] By the

---

[10] Faulkner W. *Requiem for a Nun*. New York: Random House, 1951.
[11] Experts: Iraq may have smallpox. Associated Press. 8 October 2002.

time the administration announced a vaccination plan in December 2002, the White House had narrowed the initial phase of vaccination to first responders.[12] As in 1976, however, there was no workable plan for vaccine distribution and inadequate attention to liability for vaccine makers.

In an echo of President Ford 25 years earlier, President Bush attempted to reassure the public by receiving the vaccination himself. But again, it was no use. The program ended about six months in, without any sign of smallpox, after just 38,000 of an expected 500,000 people had received the vaccine. The Institute of Medicine, in reviewing the program after the fact, found that the "program rationale was unclear," with "implementation compromised" and an "unknown effect on preparedness."[13]

A few years later, US public health officials had another chance to learn the lessons of history. In 2009, another novel influenza type—the H1N1 strain—quickly spread from Mexico to the United States. Public health leaders gave a green light to the development of a targeted vaccine. But, unlike in 1976, they publicly stated they would later decide based on the facts at hand whether to use it.

"I like the fact that they have said, 'We may change our minds,'" one expert told *The Los Angeles Times*. That expert? Dr. David Sencer, who had lost his job as director of the CDC after the 1976 swine flu crisis.[14]

Several months later, the H1N1 vaccine was found to be safe and effective, and a national vaccination campaign not only saved lives from disease but also led to a sustainable increase in influenza vaccine coverage among pregnant women.[15]

Challenge and Opportunity in Crisis

Once informed by a sense of history, public health students and practitioners should turn next to learning the four key steps of crisis response: identifying the crisis, managing the crisis, addressing communications and politics, and pivoting to long-lasting change. As a few examples illustrate, there are perils and promise all along the path of crisis management.

---

[12] Stephenson RW, Stolberg SG. Bush lays out plan on smallpox shots. *New York Times*. 14 December 2002.

[13] Baciu A. *The Smallpox Vaccination Program: Public Health in an Age of Terrorism*. Washington, DC: National Academies Press, 2005: 5.

[14] Roan S. Swine flu "debacle" of 1976 is recalled. *The Los Angeles Times*. 27 April 2009.

[15] Schnirring L. US data show higher flu vaccine uptake in kids, adults, health workers. CIDRAP News. 26 September 2013. Accessed May 31, 2017, at http://www.cidrap.umn.edu/news-perspective/2013/09/us-data-show-higher-flu-vaccine-uptake-kids-adults-health-workers.

Identifying the Crisis

In early 2014, the World Health Organization treated an Ebola outbreak in rural Guinea as no different from small outbreaks that occasionally had occurred elsewhere in Africa. Ranking the situation as a 2 on a scale of 1 to 3, the organization deferred to regional public health authorities, declining to mobilize an international response.[16]

Then the virus spread to cities. By the time that the World Health Organization realized the severity of the situation, thousands were dead, CDC Director Thomas Frieden had sounded the alarm, and Dr. Jim Kim of the World Bank had warned, "The future of the continent is on the line."[17]

Critics later pilloried the World Health Organization for an inability to recognize a global infectious catastrophe—ostensibly one of the main reasons to have an international health organization in the first place. After-action reports found that the organization "tends to adopt a reactive, rather than a proactive, response to emergencies" and "does not have a culture that supports open and critical dialogue between senior leaders and staff or that permits risk-taking or critical approaches to decisionmaking."[18] As an editorial in *The Washington Post* noted, "it was not WHO but rather Doctors without Borders, a charity, that took the early lead in warning about Ebola and battling the virus in West Africa."[19]

Managing the Crisis

As Ebola was spreading in West Africa, a different kind of crisis was brewing in the Veterans Administration (VA) in the United States. Despite ample evidence of problems facing veterans in accessing care over the previous 15 years,[20] agency leaders were unprepared for media reports that multiple VA hospitals had falsified wait times to cover up delays in treatment.[21] The Inspector General, numerous media organizations, and

---

[16] Sun L, Dennis B, Bernstein L, Achenbach J. How the world's health organizations failed to stop the Ebola disaster. *The Washington Post*. 4 October 2014.

[17] Sun L, Dennis B, Bernstein L, Achenbach J. How the world's health organizations failed to stop the Ebola disaster. *The Washington Post*. 4 October 2014.

[18] World Health Organization. Report of the Ebola Interim Assessment Panel. July 2015. Accessed May 31, 2017, at http://www.who.int/csr/resources/publications/ebola/ebola-panel-report/en/.

[19] Putting out the fire, next time. *The Washington Post*. 26 July 2015.

[20] Parlapiano A, Yourish K. Major reports and testimony on VA patient wait times. *The New York Times*. 29 May 2014.

[21] Bronstein S, Griffin G. A fatal wait: Veterans languish and die on a VA hospital's secret wait list. CNN. 23 April 2014.

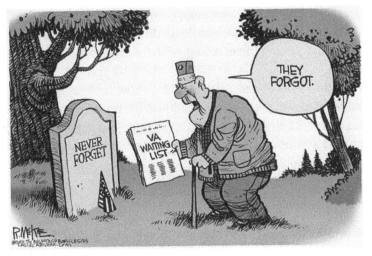

FIGURE 1.2 The Veterans Administration crisis
Courtesy of Cagle Cartoons, Inc.

multiple Congressional Committees investigated and found a culture seemingly at odds with compassionate, effective care (Figure 1.2).

As one veteran wrote in a local Alaska newspaper, "Trust is a huge issue to veterans. We do not give it easily. When we do it must be earned and maintained. Betray that and it will take years to regain that trust if ever. A lot of veterans may choose to never use VA facilities ever again because of this mess. And they are likely to be the ones in the dire need of them."[22]

Unfortunately, the VA was unable to respond to the crisis effectively. Despite the public outcry, news reports found that little was changing. The resulting firestorm, fueled by passionate advocates and veterans themselves, led to the resignation of Secretary Eric Shinseki, himself a decorated veteran.

Communication and Politics

In 2015, the city of Flint, Michigan, changed the source of municipal water without implementing appropriate controls for corrosion, leading to the leaching of lead from pipes across the city. As evidence began to mount of risks to residents, health officials missed the chance to take prompt steps to remedy the situation. To make matters worse, their communication efforts focused on providing reassurance to the public. Even after a visiting scientist from Virginia began reporting

---

[22] Grota D. VA scandal is a betrayal of our trust. *The Mat-Su Valley Frontiersman.* 16 May 2014.

high levels of lead in the water supply, officials continued to minimize the situation.[23] A spokesman attacked "dire public health advice based on some quick testing" that "could be seen as fanning political flames irresponsibly."[24]

By the time a local pediatrician held a press conference to announce her finding of elevated lead levels in children, it was too late for the public agencies involved to regain credibility. Multiple resignations followed, and the state's Attorney General has pursued criminal charges against several health officials.[25]

Pivoting to Achieve Long-Term Gains

Not all health crises end badly; health officials who recognize crises early, manage them well, and communicate well can accomplish long-sought policy change.

In 2010, the CDC and FDA quickly traced a major *Salmonella* outbreak to two large Iowa egg farms and ordered an egg recall involving—and this is not a typographical error—*half of a billion* eggs.[26] Congressional hearings revealed that FDA inspectors had found massive piles of chicken manure and extensive rodent infestation on the farm (Figure 1.3).[27] As one historian noted:

> Looking at photographs of dead chickens, insects, and manure in hen houses at the two farms associated with the outbreak, Bart Stupak (D-MI), chairman of the House Energy and Commerce Subcommittee on Oversight and Investigations, commented that the outbreak painted "a very disturbing picture of egg production in America." Energy and Commerce Chairman Henry Waxman (D-CA) went further, accusing the company and its executives of being "habitual violator[s] of basic safety standards."[28]

[23] McQuaid J. Without these whistleblowers, we may never have known the full extent of the Flint water crisis. *Smithsonian Magazine*. December 2016.

[24] Kennedy M. Lead-laced water In Flint: A step-by-step look at the makings of a crisis. National Public Radio. 20 April 2016.

[25] Michigan attorney general charges 4 more over Flint's lead-tainted water. *The Chicago Tribune*. 20 December 2016.

[26] Half a billion eggs have been recalled. CNN. 20 August 2010.

[27] Harris G. Egg producer says his business grew too quickly. *The New York Times*. 22 September 2010.

[28] Thomas CIP. *In Food We Trust: The Politics of Purity in American Food Regulation*. Lincoln: University of Nebraska Press, 2014: 188–189.

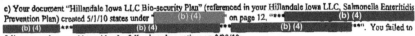

c) Your document "Hillandale Iowa LLC Bio-security Plan" (referenced in your Hillandale Iowa LLC, Salmonella Enteritidis Prevention Plan) created 5/1/10 states under " ████ (b) (4) ████ " on page 12, "*** (b) (4) ***". You failed to (b) (4) *** (b) (4) ** (b) (4) follow your plan as evidenced by the following observations on 8/20/10:

• Alden House 2 – Standing water approximately ¾ inch deep was observed on the floor adjacent to the manure pit where the foot bath was located inside the building.

• Alden House 8 – Liquid manure was observed leaking into the east section of the first floor. Plant manager reported that a water line leak occurred several weeks ago causing the manure pit to flood.

d) Your document "Hillandale II, LLP Bio-security Plan" (referenced in your Hillandale II, LLP, Salmonella Enteritidis Prevention Plan) created 5/1/10 states under " ████ (b) (4) ████ " on page 12, "*** (b) (4) ***". You failed to (b) (4) ** (b) (4) ** (b) (4) ***". You failed to follow your plan as evidenced by the following observation on 8/23/10:

• West Union House 7 - Liquid manure was observed streaming out of an approximate 6 inch gap of the east door of the manure pit. Plant manager reported a water leak had occurred.

FIGURE 1.3 The findings of the FDA's inspection of the farm responsible for contaminated eggs shocked Congress and helped lead to reform

The FDA steered the hearing, and related media attention, to underlying policy failures related to an absence of preventive controls. Moving rapidly, the agency inspected other large egg companies and released the results, keeping the issue in the news. Public disgust with the massive egg recall propelled the legislative process forward. Within a few months, Congress passed and President Obama signed the Food Safety Modernization Act, legislation that had been in the works for years. The Act authorized the FDA for the first time to establish preventive standards across the agricultural industry, what President Obama called "critically important new tools to protect our nation's food supply and keep consumers safe."[29]

In late 2012, another crisis led to fundamental changes in policy. Tennessee health officials uncovered an outbreak of meningitis associated with the use of medications compounded by a company called the New England Compounding Center.[30] Investigation revealed that the Center was manufacturing large quantities of pharmaceuticals for injection into the cerebrospinal fluid. FDA inspectors arrived on the scene and found bacteria and mold on multiple surfaces, with "greenish-black foreign matter" growing in some of the vials.[31] Public health officials rapidly traced the contaminated medications to hundreds of physician practices in

---

[29] Harris G, Neuman W. Senate passes sweeping law on food safety. *The New York Times.* 30 November 2010.

[30] Pharmaceutical compounding is an activity in which pharmacists mix ingredients together to make medications outside of the usual oversight of drug manufacturing.

[31] Walker A. Mold, bacteria found in pharmacy linked to meningitis outbreak. *The Baltimore Sun.* 26 October 2012.

more than 20 states; more than 750 people had suffered serious illnesses as a result, and 64 died.[32]

This meningitis outbreak was not the first to be tied to compounded medications, but it was the first to generate sustained national attention. Members of Congress and leading newspapers demanded accountability for the unfolding disaster. In response, FDA Commissioner Dr. Margaret Hamburg not only described the actions of her agency and multiple local and state health departments but called attention to gaps in law. She testified to Congress, "FDA's ability to take action against compounding that exceeds the bounds of traditional pharmacy compounding and poses risks to patients has been hampered by gaps and ambiguities in the law, which have led to legal challenges to FDA's authority to inspect pharmacies and take appropriate enforcement actions."[33] Hamburg then proposed a new framework that would establish much strong rules for companies making products in large quantities. This framework became the basis of the Drug Quality and Security Act, which was passed by Congress and signed by President Obama on November 27, 2013.

Crisis Strategy

Today's public health crises play out against a backdrop of a splintered media, partisan tensions, and public cynicism about government officials. This means that every mistake will be magnified and most victories soon forgotten. As Tom Nicholas has written, "It rarely occurs to the skeptics that for every terrible mistake, there are countless successes that prolong their lives."[34] This difficult situation, however, is not reason for despair.

It's a reason for strategy.

For example, by engaging the public, seeking formal input from experts, and writing compelling reports to frame a problem, health officials can manage competing interests and navigate through choppy political waters.

Health officials in crisis can also accept blame for what went wrong to maintain credibility and survive with reputations intact. This is not easy.

---

[32] CDC. Multistate outbreak of fungal meningitis and other infections—Case Count I HAI I CDC. CDC.gov. 29 October 2015. Accessed April 23, 2017, at https://www.cdc.gov/hai/outbreaks/meningitis-map-large.html.

[33] Hamburg M. Statement of Margaret A. Hamburg, M.D. Commissioner of Food and Drugs Food and Drug Administration Department of Health and Human Services before the Committee on Health, Education, Labor and Pensions. 15 November 2012. Accessed May 31, 2017, at https://www.help.senate.gov/download/2012/11/15/test-3.

[34] Nichols T. *The Death of Expertise*. New York: Oxford University Press, 2017: 24.

There can be enormous pressure to deny all responsibility, even when the facts suggest otherwise. Stepping forward to accept a share of the blame, however, may allow health officials to better position themselves and their agency for future success.

Health officials can even be strategic about using the power of a crisis to accomplish key goals. No, this is not the same as encouraging health officials to create problems to solve; that would be unethical and wrong. Rather, the opportunity is to use the tools of crisis leadership and management to elevate serious problems into urgent matters deserving attention and resources.

Think of it this way. Nobody would support a fire chief driving around the city and starting fires to call attention to inadequate fire safety standards. But what if the fire chief drove her biggest engine to the front of City Hall, blasted the sirens, unfurled the hoses, and told assembled reporters that inadequate fire safety standards were an accident waiting to happen? Well, then she might prevent a lot of fires.

My First Week

So how did I survive my first week on the job as Health Commissioner of Baltimore?

With respect to the shortage of the rabies vaccine, we reviewed the data in Baltimore and found a recent increase in the number of animals found to have rabies—an explanation for why our stocks of vaccine were running low. We quickly issued a citywide alert on rabies and changed our internal policy to reserve supplies for the uninsured. The resulting news story focused not on the woman attacked by the raccoon, but instead on the new data and how the Health Department was responding to the rabies challenge.[35] (Fortunately, the woman recovered fully.)

In response to the standoff with idealistic college students eager to feed individuals experiencing homelessness, I called their university's president and asked to bring a Health Department delegation to campus the next day to hear from the students themselves. One told us of providing food to the same set of men on the streets every week for all four years of college—more a part of her college experience, she explained, than anything else. We returned to the office and looked for a compromise. The Health Department made changes to our enforcement of the handwashing

---

[35] Roylance F. Rabies cases surge in city. *The Baltimore Sun*. 15 December 2005.

regulation and permitted the students to continue providing food to the homeless at a nearby location.

I also publicly praised the students for their community service, and they responded in kind. One was quoted as saying, "I think this is a great solution. . . . I think it's actually a step up, because they're helping us connect our food program with getting people into services through the city."[36] *The Baltimore Sun* supported our resolution of the situation,[37] and some of the students later worked with the Health Department on initiatives to end homelessness.

To keep people from freezing to death on the streets of Baltimore, we quickly reviewed data for the previous several years and found half of the deaths among the homeless happened when temperatures exceeded 25 degrees.[38] So we loosened restrictions on when to open the emergency shelter. The city's director of Homeless Services was quoted as saying the "policy change was 'wonderful,' not only for preventing deaths in the cold but also for the chance to refer more homeless people to agencies that help with drug treatment and health care."[39]

In response to the FDA's warning letter about our Institutional Review Board, I turned immediately to the city solicitor for help. Following his guidance, we set up a rapid response team that disbanded the Board altogether and signed affiliation agreements with others in the city, permitting needed research and clinical care to continue without interruption.

And, finally, in advance of the looming transition to Medicare Part D, the Health Department established a 24/7 emergency response program through local pharmacies to identify and assist low-income city residents unable to receive their essential medications. The Health Department held a press conference with the mayor to warn about the coming disruption, and, after January 1, the Health Department issued regular bulletins with data on how many people were experiencing problems. Our efforts were covered by multiple press outlets, including *The Los Angeles Times*[40] and

---

[36] Accord reached on feeding homeless. *The Baltimore Sun*. 17 December 2005.

[37] Two wrongs and a right. *The Baltimore Sun*. 18 December 2005.

[38] Hirsch A. Winter shelter relaxes criteria; After deaths of 4 homeless men, city says program can remain open at higher temperatures. *The Baltimore Sun*. 24 December 2005.

[39] Hirsch A. Winter shelter relaxes criteria; After deaths of 4 homeless men, city says program can remain open at higher temperatures. *The Baltimore Sun*. 24 December 2005.

[40] Alonso-Zaldivar R. The Nation: Baltimore goes on the alert for drug benefit snafus. *The Los Angeles Times*. 21 December 2005.

National Public Radio, which reported, "The city of Baltimore is treating the start of the program like a public health emergency."[41]

More than a decade later, I remember each of these events like they happened yesterday. These experiences not only sparked my own interest in the history, management, and strategy of crisis; they jump-started my career in public health.

---

[41] Silberner J. Baltimore takes creative tack on new drug benefit. National Public Radio. 21 December 2005.

I | History

P UBLIC HEALTH CRISES HAVE affected every community, and every health agency, in every era. One way to begin to learn from this vast history is to appreciate four iconic crises of the last century. Each of these crises defined not only the careers of many men and women in public health but also the trajectory of agencies and the health of millions of people. Each crisis also had impacts that endure to the present day. In the stories of these events, it is possible to find paradigms of crisis management to aim for—and to avoid.

Chapter 2 describes the national panic over deaths caused by the Elixir Sulfanilamide in 1937—a panic that upended the national discussion of medication safety and led to landmark legislation. Chapter 3 recounts a global calamity in 1961 involving thousands of severe birth defects caused by the medication thalidomide. The crisis sparked major changes in the oversight of medications in the United States and eventually around the world.

Not every story of crisis has a happy ending. Chapter 4 tells what happened when the federal government adopted a goal of vaccinating every American against a disease that was more imagined than real and did not adapt its plan as more evidence emerged. The swine flu debacle of 1976 still haunts vaccination policy decades later. Chapter 5 details how effective advocacy during HIV epidemic in the late 1980s caused a profound crisis in confidence for the Food and Drug Administration and the National Institutes of Health, and how these agencies responded.

1 History

2 | Elixir Sulfanilamide

Dr. Young: Were you here in Atlanta when that great chase went on?

Mr. Schiffman: Yeah. We were all sent out, most of the force, and I had occasion to go chase around in the mountains of Georgia. That's a good story.

Dr. Young: Tell us about your chase around the mountains.

Mr. Schiffman: Well, at that time, it was pretty lousy weather, raining, and the roads were pretty difficult in the mounts of Georgia at that time. And there was quite a chase to find out the locations of different people who had children who were being given this Elixir Sulfanilamide.[1]

ON OCTOBER 11, 1937, THE telephone rang at the American Medical Association offices in Chicago. On the line was the president of the Tulsa, Oklahoma, Medical Society. He explained that six area residents—including several children—had died soon after consuming a new therapy for infections marketed as the Elixir Sulfanilamide (Figure 2.1).[2] Three days later, on October 14, the Tulsa news reached a small agency inside the U.S. Department of Agriculture, the U.S. Food, Drug, and Insecticide Administration. That agency—and the field of medicine—would never be the same again.

With what historians would later call "fantastic zeal and efficiency," the FDA mobilized.[3] An inspector sent to Tulsa reported back on October 16 with details on the deaths of seven adults and two children. The gruesome autopsy report showed swollen and disfigured kidneys. Simultaneously,

---

[1] Schiffman C. Interview between John J. McManus, Retired Director of the U.S. Food and Drug Administration (FDA) Atlanta District; Clarence D. Schiffman, Retired Chemist FDA Atlanta District; and historian James Harvey Young, Emory University, 1968.

[2] Young JH. Sulfanilamide and Diethylene Glycol. Paper presented at ACS Symposium Series, No. 288: Chemistry and Modern Society: Historical Essays in Honor of Aaron J. Ihde, 1983.

[3] Jackson CO. *Food and Drug Legislation in the New Deal.* 2015th ed. Princeton, NJ: Princeton University Press, 1970: 157.

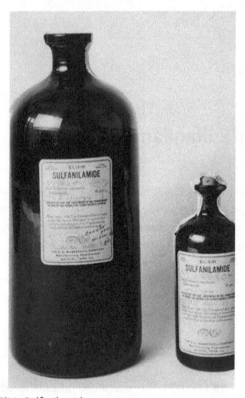

FIGURE 2.1 The Elixir Sulfanilamide

SOURCE: Food and Drug Administration
https://www.flickr.com/photos/fdaphotos/4901387552

a different team of FDA inspectors discovered that the product's manufacturer, the S.E. Massengill Company of Tennessee, had not conducted any safety testing before sale. The agency ordered the seizure of all outstanding shipments.

On October 19, the FDA directed Massengill to send out telegrams calling for the immediate return of all Elixir Sulfanilamide in distribution because of the threat to human life. The agency did not assume the telegrams would be fully successful. Using "practically the entire field force of 239 Food and Drug Administration inspectors and chemists,"[4] the agency started to track down all the remaining product itself.

It was hardly an undercover operation. On October 23, 1937, *The Washington Post* reported that "from coast to coast, in large cities like New York and backwoods communities of the South, West, and Midwest, field agents are desperately fighting against time to save lives of potential

---

[4] Jackson CO. *Food and Drug Legislation in the New Deal*. Princeton, NJ: Princeton University Press, 1970: 157.

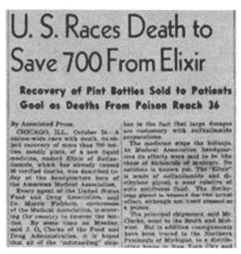

FIGURE 2.2 Associated Press coverage covered FDA's hunt for the Elixir Sulfanilamide
SOURCE: Food and Drug Administration
https://www.flickr.com/photos/fdaphotos/with/4901387552/

victims who have the elixir in their medicine cabinets."[5] Historian Daniel Carpenter noted, "Newspaper stories told of FDA officials working late nights and weekends to inform the public, of commandeering airplanes and academic chemists to search far and wide for remaining samples of the drug, and generally of a vast, nationwide operation centered in the FDA" (Figure 2.2).[6]

Within several weeks, the agency recovered all 700 bottles of the Elixir Sulfanilamide. While more than 90 people had died, the FDA's actions had saved the lives of an estimated 4,000 Americans. The FDA also discovered that the source of the problem was a deadly solvent, diethylene glycol, that had been used to suspend the medicine in solution.

Within a year of resolving the crisis, the FDA was no longer an obscure agency. Congress had passed and President Franklin D. Roosevelt signed the landmark Food, Drug, and Cosmetic Act, which, among other major steps, authorized the FDA to establish the world's first advance review for safety of medications. "The Act of 1938," Professor Carpenter has written, "stands as one of the most important regulatory statutes in American and perhaps global history."[7]

---

[5] Carpenter D. *Reputation and Power: Organizational Image and Pharmaceutical Regulation at the FDA*. Princeton, NJ: Princeton University Press, 2010: 91.

[6] Carpenter D. *Reputation and Power: Organizational Image and Pharmaceutical Regulation at the FDA*. Princeton, NJ: Princeton University Press, 2010: 91.

[7] Carpenter D. *Reputation and Power: Organizational Image and Pharmaceutical Regulation at the FDA*. Princeton, NJ: Princeton University Press, 2010: 73.

The story of the Elixir Sulfanilamide exemplifies how much in public health has been shaped by crisis. Prior to the tragedy, no member of Congress had even proposed establishing a safety review of medications before marketing. Afterwards, legislation authorizing this major step passed by overwhelming margins.

This turn of events, however, was not inevitable. Strong preparation, a well-managed response, and astute legislative strategy made all the difference in turning crisis into opportunity. If, as Louis Pasteur has famously said, chance favors the prepared mind, then the story of the Elixir Sulfanilamide shows that crisis favors the prepared agency.

The FDA was only a few decades old when the first reports of deaths from the Elixir Sulfanilamide arrived. The agency traces its origins to the mid-1800s, to a small office called the Bureau of Chemistry in the U.S. Department of Agriculture. Its first prominent leader was Harvey Wiley, a man so devoted to public health protection that he would feed toxins to his staff at lunch and record their reactions, under a sign that stated, "None but the brave can eat the fare."[8] The Bureau focused its attention on risks to consumers in the food and drug supply.

This was no small task. At that time, hundreds of companies sold popular "patent medications," which were mixes of undisclosed ingredients commonly advertised as miraculous fixes for cancer, diabetes, or—to make it simple—every medical problem, at once. For example, Wm. R. Adams Microbe Killer was sold as a "germ, bacteria, or fungus destroyer," with the promise that it "cures all diseases."[9] Dr. King's New Discovery was described in advertisements as "the greatest cure for cough and colds . . . the King of all throat and lung remedies."[10] The Johnson Remedy Company promised "cancer can be cured . . . no matter how serious your case may be, no matter what treatment you have tried, no matter how many operations you have had."[11]

By the turn of the 20th century, these deceptions began to catch up to patient medication manufacturers. In 1906, the magazine *Collier's* published

---

[8] Junod S. The Poison Squad and the advent of food and drug regulation. *FDA Consumer*. November–December 2002. The article quotes the chorus from the "Song of the Poison Squad"—"O, they may get over it but they'll never look the same, That kind of bill of fare would drive most men insane. Next week he'll give them mothballs, a la Newburgh or else plain; O, they may get over it but they'll never look the same."

[9] Wm. Radam's Microbe Killer cures all diseases. *Galveston Daily News*. 5 November 1990, 3.

[10] The Pure Food and Drugs Act. Hearings before the Committee on Interstate and Foreign Commerce. House of Representatives. Washington, DC: Government Printing Office, 1912.

[11] The Pure Food and Drugs Act. Hearings before the Committee on Interstate and Foreign Commerce. House of Representatives. Washington, DC: Government Printing Office, 1912.

a long exposé describing these products as "palatable poison for the poor."[12] It was the Progressive Era, a time when there was broad national support for establishing a core set of regulations to oversee the private sector. In response to growing recognition of the dangers of the market for therapies, Congress passed and President Theodore Roosevelt signed the Pure Food and Drugs Act of 1906. This law required manufacturers to list key ingredients and gave some authority to act against mislabeled products to the agency that would soon be named the FDA. However, the new law only provided for limited enforcement authority and minimal fines, and it did not permit review of medications for safety before marketing.

Over the next several decades, the FDA became increasingly frustrated with its own impotence. For example, the agency pursued charges against the manufacturer of "Cuforhedake Brane Fude"—on the obvious grounds that it was being marketed misleadingly as a brain food that would cure headaches. (It turned out the remedy's main ingredient was alcohol.) But despite the fact the product had earned millions in sales, the agency only succeeded in assessing $700 in fines.[13] The historian Charles O. Jackson told the story of the B & M External Remedy:

> B & M was originally a horse liniment, composed mainly of ammonia, turpentine, water, and egg. It came to be offered to the public as a treatment for human tuberculosis, pneumonia, and other diseases. The Food and Drug Administration collected records of sixty-four fatalities laid to the direct or indirect effects of B& M, as part of a legal case against its producers. Even at this, it took FDA ten years . . . to prosecute the case successfully.[14]

The manufacturer of the useless product Banbar continued marketing to individuals suffering from diabetes, even though the world's first effective treatment, insulin, had recently been discovered. Banbar was featured when the FDA's information officer Ruth Lamb began a national advocacy campaign to support new authority for the agency. As part of the campaign, Lamb created a traveling display called the Chamber of Horrors. The display presented copies of testimonials written by patients about their successful treatment with Banbar—alongside copies, dated several weeks to months later, of the very same patients' death certificates. After

---

[12] The patent medicine trust: Palatable poison for the poor. *Collier's: The National Weekly,* 1905.
[13] Carpenter D. *Reputation and Power: Organizational Image and Pharmaceutical Regulation at the FDA.* Princeton, NJ: Princeton University Press, 2010: 80.
[14] Jackson CO. *Food and Drug Legislation in the New Deal.* Princeton, NJ: Princeton University Press, 1970: 7.

the patent medicine industry claimed the display might violate prohibitions on agencies lobbying Congress, Lamb published a book under her own name titled *American Chamber of Horrors* about the weaknesses of the 1906 law.[15]

Following the election of President Franklin D. Roosevelt in 1932, FDA Commissioner Walter Campbell tried to push for more authority to protect the nation from unsafe drugs. But for the next five years, the agency failed repeatedly. The FDA's main ally in Congress was New York Senator Royal Copeland, a homeopathic physician who had served as New York Health Commissioner during the influenza pandemic of 1918. However, Senator Copeland's influence was limited because he opposed President Roosevelt's New Deal. In fact, in the fall of 1934, the president's political advisor declined to support Copeland's re-election.[16] In 1935, allies of the patent medicine industry succeeded in attaching an amendment to Senator Copeland's bill that would send most authority over medications to the Federal Trade Commission. The bill was then killed in the House of Representatives. By mid-1937, Senator Copeland was about to give up.[17]

At that very moment, however, salesmen began asking the S.E. Massengill company to develop a liquid formulation of the new sulfanilamide drug, which in a class of early antimicrobial treatments showed some effectiveness against a range of infections, including gonorrhea, septicemia, and sore throat. Historian Charles O. Jackson noted that "American physicians were quick to recognize the far-reaching effects of the drug, and by 1937 its use had grown to tremendous proportions."[18] A liquid formulation would expand the drug's use in children and be available to patients who did not wish to swallow tablets.

Making such a product, however, required finding a solution that the chemical could be dissolved in, known as a solvent. The company's chemist, Harold Cole Watkins, experimented with many solvents before discovering one that seemed perfect: diethylene glycol. The company's laboratory assessed the solution for appearance, smell, and taste—but not

---

[15] FDA. Ruth DeForest Lamb: FDA's first chief educational officer. 1 March 2013. Accessed May 29, 2017, at https://www.fda.gov/AboutFDA/WhatWeDo/History/ucm341860.htm.

[16] Jackson CO. *Food and Drug Legislation in the New Deal.* Princeton, NJ: Princeton University Press, 1970: 63.

[17] Carpenter D. *Reputation and Power: Organizational Image and Pharmaceutical Regulation at the FDA.* Princeton, NJ: Princeton University Press, 2010.

[18] Jackson CO. *Food and Drug Legislation in the New Deal.* Princeton, NJ: Princeton University Press, 1970: 152.

for safety. On August 28, 1937, Massengill began to manufacture what would turn out to be 240 gallons of product.[19]

Then: Illness. Death. Crisis. A vigorous agency response. Even as the FDA scrambled to send agents around the country, FDA Commissioner Campbell began to make the case that a new law was needed. This case built directly on the groundwork previously established by the agency.

One of Campbell's major arguments: The Elixir Sulfanilamide was illegal only because of a marketing technicality: The term "elixir" was reserved for products that contained alcohol, but the sulfanilamide product lacked this ingredient. Only this thin justification—and not anything to do with the injuries or deaths—made it possible for the agency to take any action to protect the public at all. In an early press release issued October 19, Campbell called for a government licensing system as the only way to prevent another tragedy.[20] He notified Senator Copeland that existing legislative proposals were now insufficient and new provisions needed to be added. He also began to lobby newspaper editors to take up the cause.

A broad coalition emerged to press for legislative change. The group included the American Medical Association, whose journal editor Dr. Morris Fishbein noted on October 23 that the Elixir Sulfanilamide was "not standardized by any reliable agency."[21] It also included the League of Women Voters, whose president Marguerite M. Wells wrote on October 28 that the crisis demonstrated "the need for federal legislation ensuring a governmental check on such products before they are distributed to a helpless public."[22]

Two weeks later, Secretary of Agriculture Henry A. Wallace sent a devastating report to Congress on the Sulfanilamide situation. Prepared by the FDA, and also released to the public, the report told the story of the tragedy in heartbreaking detail and then pointed directly to a solution: premarket review of medications for safety. The first page stated: "Before the 'elixir' was put on the market, it was tested by the firm for flavor but not for its effect on human life. The existing Food and Drugs Act does not require that new drugs be tested before they are placed for sale."[23] As Professor

---

[19] Jackson CO. *Food and Drug Legislation in the New Deal*. Princeton, NJ: Princeton University Press, 1970: 152.

[20] Carpenter D. *Reputation and Power: Organizational Image and Pharmaceutical Regulation at the FDA*. Princeton, NJ: Princeton University Press, 2010.

[21] Carpenter D. *Reputation and Power: Organizational Image and Pharmaceutical Regulation at the FDA*. Princeton, NJ: Princeton University Press, 2010.

[22] Carpenter D. *Reputation and Power: Organizational Image and Pharmaceutical Regulation at the FDA*. Princeton, NJ: Princeton University Press, 2010: 93.

[23] Wallace HA. A report on Elixir Sulfanilamide-Massengill. 16 November 1937. Washington, DC: Government Printing Office, 1937: 1.

Carpenter noted: "Translation: with a pre-market review process, none of this would have happened."[24]

The report included new details, including how the FDA interviewed about 200 company salesmen to account for their samples. It told the story of how hard it had been for the agency to find remaining doses of the poison. In one case, for example, a woman initially claimed to an FDA inspector she had destroyed her medication, before clarifying that she "simply threw the bottle out the window into an alley." The report noted, "The inspector found the bottle unbroken, still containing ample 'elixir' to kill any child intrigued to swallow its pink, sweet, aromatic liquid."[25]

The report culminated in a previously undisclosed letter from Mrs. Maise Nidiffer to President Roosevelt about the death of her six-year-old daughter Joan from the Elixir Sulfanilamide. Mrs. Nidiffer wrote:

> All that is left to us is the caring for of that little grave. Even the memory of her is mixed with sorrow for we can see her little body tossing to and fro and hear that little voice screaming with pain and it seems as though it would drive me insane . . . Tonight, President Roosevelt, as you enjoy your little grandchildren of whom we read about, it is my plea that you will take steps to prevent such sales of drugs that will take little lives and leave such suffering behind and such a bleak outlook on the future as I have tonight.[26]

The report's two final sections were titled "Limitations of the Law" and "Recommendations for Legislation." These sections put the tragedy in larger context: "While the 'elixir' incident has been spectacular and has received much publicity . . . it is but a repetition of what has frequently happened in the past in the marketing of such dangerous drugs." The report called for holding on distribution of new drugs "until experimental and clinical tests have shown them to be safe for use." The report stated: "It is the Department's view that no other form of control will effectively safeguard the public from the dangers of premature distribution of new drugs."[27]

---

[24] Carpenter D. *Reputation and Power: Organizational Image and Pharmaceutical Regulation at the FDA*. Princeton, NJ: Princeton University Press, 2010: 97.
[25] Wallace HA. A report on Elixir Sulfanilamide-Massengill. 16 November 1937. Washington, DC: Government Printing Office, 1937: 6.
[26] Wallace HA. A report on Elixir Sulfanilamide-Massengill. 16 November 1937. Washington, DC: Government Printing Office, 1937: 8.
[27] Wallace HA. A report on Elixir Sulfanilamide-Massengill. 16 November 1937. Washington, DC: Government Printing Office, 1937: 10.

The Department of Agriculture's report on the Elixir Sulfanilamide stands as a classic to this day. At the time, it sparked a national demand for a new food and drug law. It led Hollywood to create two short films, *Permit to Kill* and *G-Men of Science*, that told the story of what happened and ended with calls for change. When the Massengill company wrote to Congress in November 1937 denying that it had broken any law, the letter quickly became yet another exhibit in the case for reform. Historian John Jackson reports that on the premarket review provisions of the bill, "There was essentially no debate." While one senator "lamely brought to the attention of his colleagues the fact that objections had been raised to the bill," Senator Copeland "commented curtly that 'there are objections, and there will be objections from now to the end of time, but, so far as I can judge, the bill is in such form that it is safe to pass it.' "[28] In the space of a few years, a major expansion of FDA authority had gone from impossible to unstoppable. Key provisions included not only the establishment of premarket review for safety, but also a requirement for directions for safe use and the prohibition of false therapeutic claims.

The FDA's robust response to crisis, and its ability to pivot seamlessly from saving lives to demanding action, were essential to pushing the Food, Drug, and Cosmetic Act into law. Historian Charles O. Jackson noted that the crisis "reduced the number of legislators willing to stand adamantly for the interests of industry" and "for the first time really brought a heated public demand for legislation."[29] Professor Carpenter stated:

> Without the image of elixir sulfanilamide that an ungoverned market would kill, without the idea that an agency capable of governing that market had removed the deadly elixir from American society, and without the idea that the same organization could prevent another elixir tragedy by its power to deny market entry to new drugs unless their safety had been

[28] Carpenter D. *Reputation and Power: Organizational Image and Pharmaceutical Regulation at the FDA.* Princeton, NJ: Princeton University Press, 2010: 170. Senator Copeland's leadership was essential for the passage of the Food, Drug, and Cosmetic Act. Unfortunately, he died just a week before President Roosevelt signed the bill into law. Jackson CO. *Food and Drug Legislation in the New Deal.* Princeton, NJ: Princeton University Press, 1970: 200.

[29] Jackson CO. *Food and Drug Legislation in the New Deal.* Princeton, NJ: Princeton University Press, 1970: 218.

demonstrated—without these lessons, the faces of regulatory power would not have materialized as they did.

The experience of the Elixir Sulfanilamide led FDA to gain the ability to enforce basic standards for safety. But clear authority to review medications for effectiveness—another core standard—had to wait for another crisis.

3 | Thalidomide

F OR A STORY OF TRAGEDY followed by an effective policy response, it is hard to beat the case of the Elixir Sulfanilamide. Under the national spotlight, a fledgling agency took center stage, prevented the deaths of thousands of Americans, and persuaded Congress to pass landmark legislation.

It was not happenstance. FDA leaders had spent years honing the argument and advising the public that the nation's laws on drugs were inadequate. When the crisis hit, the agency wasted no time or expense sending hundreds of inspectors around the country, in full view of the nation's media. Nor did the agency hesitate before demanding new legal authority to protect the country.

One lesson of the Elixir Sulfanilamide crisis is that public health leaders can achieve policy success by spotting an unfolding tragedy, stepping in as the hero, and then pointing out what would have avoided the problem.

But that's not the only path to progress. The FDA would soon find that another opportunity lies in stopping untold harm in the first place—as long as the agency gets the credit.

In 1962, 24 years after the passage of the Food, Drug, and Cosmetic Act of 1938, the nation again found itself transfixed by a crisis caused by a medication, although in this case the actual harm mostly occurred overseas. That's because the FDA never approved this medication—thalidomide—for use in the United States.

Again, the FDA's actions earned the agency the gratitude of a nation. Again, Congress responded by granting the agency new legal powers this time through amendments to the 1938 law that provided "commanding new authorities,"[1] including the unprecedented power to require medications to be proven effective before sale.

---

[1] Carpenter D. *Reputation and Power: Organizational Image and Pharmaceutical Regulation at the FDA.* Princeton, NJ: Princeton University Press, 2010: 229.

Prevention has been called the dog that doesn't bark. Indeed, the work of keeping people healthy is not nearly as exciting as the work of firefighters battling blazes, police officers racing down the street, or surgeons rescuing people from the brink of death. Yet in the case of thalidomide, the FDA somehow found a way to make sure that every American family realized how close the nation came to disaster. And the key to success turned out to be a deliberate decision to highlight the role of a single person, FDA scientist Dr. Frances Kelsey, and how she exemplified the agency's mission to protect the country.

The story of thalidomide also illustrates again how preparation and strategy can lead to progress that otherwise would have been impossible.

In the years after the Elixir Sulfanilamide episode, as the FDA greatly expanded its capacity to review medications for safety, the agency became concerned about the risks posed by ineffective products. Enforcement was on the upswing, and industry publications began to report that the agency was targeting "medical quacks and frauds."[2] The FDA began to press the point that it was impossible to understand the safety of a medication without also considering whether the medication actually worked. After all, a risk of death could be tolerable for a drug that saved lives but not for one that did not help patients at all.

For their part, however, companies argued in court that existing law only provided for a safety review prior to marketing—prompting FDA officials to consider the need for new legislation.

Meanwhile, on September 12, 1960, Cincinnati manufacturer William S. Merrell Company filed an application with the FDA to market a new drug in the United States called thalidomide.

Thalidomide was first synthesized in a West German pharmaceutical lab in 1953. When given to humans, the drug led to significant sedation but without the risk of overdose seen with barbiturates (which were then commonly prescribed). In 1958, West Germany permitted thalidomide to be sold over the counter for a variety of ailments, including for nausea in pregnant women. In fact, thalidomide was marketed as particularly safe during pregnancy. Within a couple years, the drug would be sold in 46 countries.

Empowered by the 1938 law, the FDA required the Merrell Company to submit data on safety approving thalidomide. The agency's reviewer,

---

[2] Carpenter D. *Reputation and Power: Organizational Image and Pharmaceutical Regulation at the FDA*. Princeton, NJ: Princeton University Press, 2010: 199.

Dr. Francis Kelsey, was a pediatrician and pharmacologist from South Dakota on her first drug review assignment (Box 3.1).

For several months, Dr. Kelsey made a series of requests for information to the manufacturer, covering such topics as the side effect of peripheral neuritis and safety during pregnancy. She consulted with others at the agency, including her husband (who was also a pharmacologist) about major errors in the application.[3] She referenced the minimal evidence of benefit of the medication as a reason for wanting to be particularly vigilant.

Dr. Kelsey was not convinced by the company's responses to her inquiries. A year after the application was submitted, the FDA had made no decision, and Merrell executives began to express their frustration. Company leaders reached out to senior leaders at the FDA to complain of "delay after delay after delay."[4] They pointed to the wide use and apparent safety in European markets. In September 1961, the company pressed its case at the agency for approval in time to release the medication in time for the Christmas holiday.[5]

But Dr. Kelsey and her colleagues still refused. And then, on November 30, 1961, a Merrell representative called the FDA with the news that the company had withdrawn thalidomide from the market in West Germany. The reason for this action, he explained, was a theoretical concern about a possible link between the drug's use in pregnancy and a severe birth defect known as phocomelia—manifested by the total absence of arms and legs. Until this issue was resolved, Merrell asked that its application remain on hold.

Little happened at the FDA on thalidomide for the next five months. Then, in March 1962, Merrell withdrew its application for the medication altogether. In April, a Johns Hopkins University pediatrician, Dr. Helen Taussig, called FDA officials to tell them of a recent trip to Europe, where she found the evidence linking thalidomide to birth defects to be quite strong. Indeed, thousands of German babies were now being born with phocomelia, which previously had been vanishingly rare. On April 11, a few news stories reported Dr. Taussig's concerns about thalidomide. The

---

[3] In one case, her husband, F. Ellis Kelsey, found it absurd that Merrell had compared the dosage for thalidomide by weight with a dosage for another drug without adjusting for the size of the specific molecules. "Since this is an elementary concept of pharmacology I cannot believe this to be honest incompetence," he wrote. Carpenter D. *Reputation and Power: Organizational Image and Pharmaceutical Regulation at the FDA*. Princeton, NJ: Princeton University Press, 2010: 220.

[4] Carpenter D. *Reputation and Power: Organizational Image and Pharmaceutical Regulation at the FDA*. Princeton, NJ: Princeton University Press, 2010: 225.

[5] McFayden, RE. Thalidomide in America: A brush with tragedy. *Clio Medica*. 1976;11(2):79–93.

BOX 3.1 FRANCES KELSEY, THE HEROINE OF THE FDA

by Grace Mandel

Dr. Frances Kelsey, a remarkable woman with a remarkable career, became known not only for her contributions to the thalidomide case but also for breaking barriers for women in science.

Born as Frances Oldham in 1914, Dr. Kelsey graduated with a bachelor's degree in biochemistry from McGill University in 1934.[1] She immediately began looking for work but was unable to find a job due to the Great Depression. She enrolled in a master's program in the pharmacology department.

With encouragement from a mentor, Dr. Kelsey sent a letter applying to study for a PhD with a new professor at the University of Chicago. In her autobiographical reflections, Kelsey commented on the reply that she received:

> It started out, "Dear Mr. Oldham," and my conscience tweaked me a bit. I knew that men were the preferred commodity in those days. Should I write and explain that Frances with an "e" is female and with an "i" is male? . . . to this day, I do not know if my name had been Elizabeth or Mary Jane, whether I would have gotten that first big step up. My professor at Chicago to his dying day would never admit one way or another.[2]

Frances Kelsey received her PhD in 1938. Dr. Kelsey's first introduction to work with the FDA was as a graduate student. She was part of the pharmacology team that identified diethylene glycol as the toxic substance in the elixir sulfanilamide. This experience gave her a sense of the harm that could be done by unsafe medications. She graduated from the University of Chicago School of Medicine in 1950.

A decade later, after her husband received a job offer at the National Institutes of Health, Dr. Kelsey moved to Washington and began working at the FDA as a medical officer. She later noted, "It was very difficult in those days to get people to work as medical officers in the government. The pay was very low compared to what a physician could earn elsewhere." For her first assignment, she was given the thalidomide application because it was supposed to be straightforward. She said, "I was the new one there and pretty green, so my supervisors decided, 'Well, this is a very easy one. There will be no problems with sleeping pills.' So that is how I happened to get the application."[3]

---

[1] Kelsey F. Autobiographical reflections. U.S. Food and Drug Administration, 1993. Accessed June 29, 2017, at https://www.fda.gov/downloads/AboutFDA/WhatWeDo/History/OralHistories/SelectedOralHistoryTranscripts/UCM406132.pdf

[2] Kelsey F. Autobiographical reflections. U.S. Food and Drug Administration, 1993. Accessed June 29, 2017, at https://www.fda.gov/downloads/AboutFDA/WhatWeDo/History/OralHistories/SelectedOralHistoryTranscripts/UCM406132.pdf

[3] Kelsey F. Autobiographical reflections. U.S. Food and Drug Administration, 1993. Accessed June 29, 2017, at https://www.fda.gov/downloads/AboutFDA/WhatWeDo/History/OralHistories/SelectedOralHistoryTranscripts/UCM406132.pdf

next month, Dr. Taussig testified before the House of Representatives, but again, without significant national attention.

At the start of the summer of 1962, the story of thalidomide had barely made a blip in the United States. But it did catch the attention of Sen. Estes Kefauver of Tennessee. A former vice presidential candidate with national ambitions, Senator Kefauver had for years been trying to strengthen drug laws in the United States. He was not having much success, with the pharmaceutical industry blocking him at each turn and President Kennedy and his advisers not confident in a path to legislative success.[6] After hearing the story of thalidomide, Senator Kefauver and his staff hatched a plan to jump-start their stalled legislation.

Their idea was to focus on Dr. Kelsey herself. She had, after all, blocked the approval of a drug that was causing devastating effects in Europe. Her expertise, her character, and her courage had saved thousands of US babies. The senator's staff called *The Washington Post*, and reporter Morton Mintz interviewed Dr. Kelsey and published a front-page story on July 15, 1962.

The headline read: "'Heroine' of FDA Keeps Bad Drug Off Market." The article began, "This is the story of how the skepticism and stubbornness of a Government physician prevented what could have been an appalling American tragedy, the birth of hundreds or indeed thousands of armless and legless children."[7]

Mintz wrote about how "Dr. Frances Oldham Kelsey, a Food and Drug Administration medical officer" refused "to be hurried into approving an application for marketing a new drug."[8] While noting that "Dr. Kelsey's tenacity . . . was upheld by her superiors, all the way," Mintz detailed how she resisted multiple direct and indirect attempts to convince her to approve the drug before she had appropriate evidence in hand. He concluded, "For 20 years she taught pharmacology. She knows the dangers, and she has not the slightest intention of forgetting them."[9]

An "avalanche of publicity"[10] followed Mintz's story. Every major daily newspaper recounted how a heroic drug reviewer saved thousands of babies. *Time Magazine* covered the "Thalidomide Disaster." *Good Housekeeping* wrote about "Dr. Kelsey's Stubborn Triumph," *Life Magazine* described the

[6] Carpenter D. *Reputation and Power: Organizational Image and Pharmaceutical Regulation at the FDA*. Princeton, NJ: Princeton University Press, 2010: 236.

[7] Mintz M. "Heroine" of FDA keeps bad drug off market. *The Washington Post*. 15 July 1962.

[8] Mintz M. "Heroine" of FDA keeps bad drug off market. *The Washington Post*. 15 July 1962.

[9] Mintz M. "Heroine" of FDA keeps bad drug off market. *The Washington Post*. 15 July 1962.

[10] Carpenter D. *Reputation and Power: Organizational Image and Pharmaceutical Regulation at the FDA*. Princeton, NJ: Princeton University Press, 2010: 242.

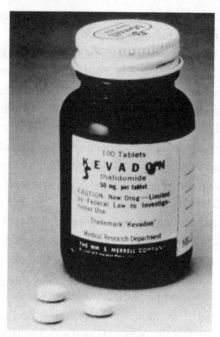

FIGURE 3.1 A bottle of thalidomide distributed for investigational purposes
SOURCE: United States Food and Drug Administration
https://www.flickr.com/photos/fdaphotos/with/4901387552/

"Woman Doctor Who Would Not Be Hurried," *Readers Digest* announced, "Doctor Kelsey Said No," and *Catholic Standard* introduced "Dr. Kelsey, Heroine." The *New York Herald Tribune* stated, "Every American family stands in debt to Frances Kelsey."[11]

In late July 1962, the FDA disclosed that some thalidomide had actually made it into the United States. Even though its application had not been approved for general marketing, Merrell had distributed the drug for research purposes to more than 1,000 physicians, some of whom had given free samples to patients (Figure 3.1). As a result, FDA explained, some remaining bottles of thalidomide might still be in medicine cabinets across the country. The resulting firestorm of attention was so great that, on August 1, President John F. Kennedy took the opportunity to address the nation and call for a stronger drug law. He stated:

Recent events in the country and abroad concerning the effects of a new sedative called thalidomide emphasize again the urgency of providing

---

[11] Carpenter D. *Reputation and Power: Organizational Image and Pharmaceutical Regulation at the FDA*. Princeton, NJ: Princeton University Press, 2010: 247.

additional protection to American consumers from harmful or worthless drug products.

Kennedy added that "the Food and Drug Administration has had nearly two hundred people working on this, and every doctor, every hospital, every nurse has been notified." He personally expressed his thanks to Dr. Kelsey.[12]

Thalidomide quickly became a national focus of attention. In the wake of the press conference, "the agenda, content, and emotion of pharmaceutical politics changed,"[13] and Senator Kefauver's efforts to get additional authority for the FDA caught fire. Administration aides helped redraft the bill, adding back provisions that had been taken out for lack of support.

Some wondered why there was any need to change the law; after all, the FDA had done a pretty good job of protecting the public under the existing statute. At one point in the ensuing Congressional debate, New York Senator Jacob Javits noted, "It may not be necessary to pass such legislation . . . indeed the Kelsey case may show the present system is working pretty well and that legislation may not be needed."[14] Senator Kefauver and the FDA responded that stronger laws that required a demonstration of the effectiveness of medications would help the agency avoid such close calls in the future. In the wake of averted tragedy, and of growing admiration for the agency, there was no stopping the bill's momentum in Congress.

On October 10, 1962, President Kennedy—with invited guest Dr. Frances Kelsey standing over his shoulder—signed the 1962 amendments to the Food, Drug and Cosmetic Act. For the first time, the law imposed strong controls over the use of medications for research activities during the preapproval phase. The law also required that drugs be proven effective prior to marketing on the basis of "adequate and well-controlled studies." This single phrase would transform clinical investigation and the pharmaceutical industry in the United States and around the world. Indeed, evidence of effectiveness would usher in what many would call a golden age for the pharmaceutical industry and clinical medicine.

---

[12] Dr. Kelsey receives gold medal from Kennedy at White House. *The New York Times.* 7 August 1962.
[13] Carpenter D. *Reputation and Power: Organizational Image and Pharmaceutical Regulation at the FDA.* Princeton, NJ: Princeton University Press, 2010: 256.
[14] Carpenter D. *Reputation and Power: Organizational Image and Pharmaceutical Regulation at the FDA.* Princeton, NJ: Princeton University Press, 2010: 255.

These changes would not have happened but for thalidomide. As Professor Carpenter writes in his seminal history of the FDA, "There are moments even in American politics when heaven and earth seem to align, when the felt pressure for legislation produces quick, consensual action that subsumes and elides permanent disagreements. Thalidomide created one of those moments."[15] Thirty years later, more than two-thirds of US residents over the age of 45 could correctly recall the story of thalidomide.[16]

The thalidomide crisis shows that the impetus for policy change requires more than a tragedy. Change depends not only on the number of people affected by a problem but also on the political context, on social expectations, and on the readiness of an agency to lead. In 1962, change was made possible by an enterprising senator and a health agency ready to seize on a moment of national focus.[17]

Indeed, a stark contrast can be drawn between what happened in the United States and the fate of pharmaceutical regulation in West Germany—a country that in the end experienced nearly 10,000 severe birth defects as a result of thalidomide. The situation in West Germany might seem more likely to lead to public outrage and a demand for stronger safety standards. And there was indeed public outrage. But the focus in West Germany was on blame, and litigation over the catastrophe persisted for the next decade. Only in 1971 did West Germany adopt a law modeled on the 1962 US law.

As for Dr. Kelsey, she remained a revered figure in American culture. In 1962, she became the first woman to receive the Distinguished Civilian Service Award, the nation's highest honor for government service (Figure 3.2). Now, every year, the FDA awards the Kelsey Award for Excellence and Courage in Protecting Public Health.

---

[15] Carpenter D. *Reputation and Power: Organizational Image and Pharmaceutical Regulation at the FDA*. Princeton, NJ: Princeton University Press, 2010: 230.

[16] Carpenter D. *Reputation and Power: Organizational Image and Pharmaceutical Regulation at the FDA*. Princeton, NJ: Princeton University Press, 2010: 255.

[17] Unfortunately, Senator Kefauver died of a ruptured aortic aneurysm in 1963, soon after the passage of the 1962 Amendments.

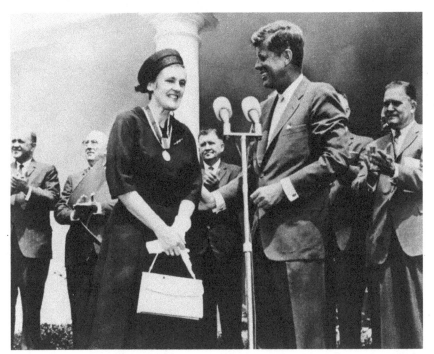

FIGURE 3.2 Dr. Frances Kelsey receives the Distinguished Civilian Service Award from President John F. Kennedy in 1962

Courtesy John F. Kennedy Library
https://www.jfklibrary.org/Asset-Viewer/Archives/JFKWHP-AR7400-C.aspx

With the passage of major legislation in 1938 and again in 1962, the FDA in the 20th century exemplified the power of agency preparation and crisis response to advance the public health. Little more than a decade later, however, the U.S. Public Health Service would find out that a poor response to crisis could have quite the opposite effect.

4 | The Swine Flu of 1976

I N LATE 1979, MORE THAN 40 million Americans sat down every Sunday evening to watch *60 Minutes*, the CBS news magazine program that was the top-rated television show in America. This was an era before cable television, before the Internet—and even before most Americans had the ability to record shows to watch later. More than one in four US households with televisions tuned in to *60 Minutes* each week.[1]

On November 4, 1979, reporter Mike Wallace began a segment of the broadcast:

> The flu season is upon us. Which type will we worry about this year, and what kind of shots will we be told to take? Remember the swine flu scare of 1976? That was the year the US government told us all that swine flu could turn out to be a killer that could spread across the nation, and Washington decided that every man, woman and child in the nation should get a shot to prevent a nationwide outbreak, a pandemic.
>
> Well, 46 million of us obediently took the shot, and now 4,000 Americans are claiming damages from Uncle Sam amounting to three and a half billion dollars because of what happened when they took that shot. By far the greatest number of the claims—two-thirds of them—are for neurological damage, or even death, allegedly triggered by the flu shot.[2]

For the next 20 minutes, Wallace lambasted the Centers for Disease Control and Prevention (CDC) and the U.S. Department of Health and Human

---

[1] CBS. *60 Minutes: Milestones*. 20 August 1999. Accessed May 29, 2017, at http://www.cbsnews.com/news/60-minutes-milestones/.
[2] CBS. *60 Minutes*. 4 November 1979.

Services (HHS) for mishandling the "swine flu" crisis of 1976. He told the tragic stories of individuals suffering alleged neurological complications from the vaccine recommended by the federal government. He peppered the former CDC director, Dr. Jeffrey Sencer, with questions about when the agency became aware of the potential for serious side effects.

And then, Wallace twisted the knife. He referenced "America's sweetheart," the popular actress Mary Tyler Moore. Brandishing a copy of an internal memo, the reporter alleged the CDC had planned to tell the public that Moore was one of "many important persons" who had received the vaccine. Once Sencer admitted that he did not know if the CDC had the permission to use her name, the show cut to an interview with the actress.

WALLACE: Mary, did you take a swine flu shot?

MOORE: No, I did not.

WALLACE: Did you give them permission to use your name saying that you had or were going to?

MOORE: Absolutely not. Never did.

WALLACE: Did you ask your own doctor about taking the swine flu shot?

MOORE: Yes, and at the time he thought it might be a good idea. But I resisted it, because I was leery of having the symptoms that sometimes go with that kind of inoculation.

WALLACE: So you didn't?

MOORE: No, I didn't.

WALLACE: Have you spoken to your doctor since?

MOORE: Yes.

WALLACE: And?

MOORE: He's delighted that I didn't take that shot.

Decades later, anti-vaccine activists would re-post the video and its transcript to demonstrate the incompetence of government agencies and to provide a rationale to resist vaccination.

The story of the 1976 swine flu crisis is one of failed judgment and management. The fiasco certainly did not help President Ford's failed campaign for the presidency that year. More significantly, the swine flu crisis was a self-inflicted wound to vaccination efforts that has yet to fully heal.

What in the world happened?

The story began in January 1976, at the Fort Dix US military base in New Jersey. A severe respiratory illness struck the camp, and one young soldier died. Local health officials conducting routine influenza surveillance came across several viral samples that could not be identified and sent them to the CDC. Soon after, the CDC lab reported finding a new influenza virus type resembling one usually found in pigs. The news of a "swine flu" rocketed across the agency.[3]

Sencer and other CDC leaders naturally wondered whether the new virus could reflect a genetic shift that could evade the human immune system and cause hundreds of thousands, if not millions, of deaths. It was not an entirely theoretical fear. The public health officials were well aware of what happened in 1918, when a new type of influenza had caused a global pandemic and killed millions.

CDC staff worked around the clock to analyze as much data as they could find. Then, on Saturday, February 14, Sencer convened a meeting to receive a full briefing about the Fort Dix situation, with senior officials from the National Institutes of Health, the Food and Drug Administration (FDA), and the Public Health Service giving up their Valentine's Day to attend.[4] As Professors Richard Neustadt and Harvey Fineberg would later observe in their landmark book *The Swine Flu Affair*, "The question at once became whether . . . human cases were the first appearance of an incipient pandemic or a fluke of some kind, a limited transfer to a few humans of what remained and animal disease which would not thrive in people."[5]

The group agreed to gather more data before issuing a statement to the public, but Sencer, fearing the news would leak out, called a press conference to explain what was happening. This had the effect of adding gasoline to the fire of growing concern. The next day's *New York Times* read, "The possibility was raised today that the virus that caused the greatest world epidemic of influenza in modern history—the pandemic of 1918–1919—may have returned."[6]

Meanwhile, CDC officials were learning more about the situation. About a dozen recruits had fallen ill from the new virus, with just the one death; several hundred had been infected but experienced no symptoms. This was not much evidence to go on, but an unusual deadline loomed. Every March, the federal government made the decision about which strains of the influenza virus would be covered in the fall's flu vaccine.

[3] Neustadt R, Fineberg H. *The Swine Flu Affair: Decision-Making on a Slippery Disease*. Washington, DC: National Academies Press, 1978: Chapter 1.

[4] Neustadt R, Fineberg H. *The Swine Flu Affair: Decision-Making on a Slippery Disease*. Washington, DC: National Academies Press, 1978: Chapter 1.

[5] Neustadt R, Fineberg H. *The Swine Flu Affair: Decision-Making on a Slippery Disease*. Washington, DC: National Academies Press, 1978: Chapter 1.

[6] Neustadt R, Fineberg H. *The Swine Flu Affair: Decision-Making on a Slippery Disease*. Washington, DC: National Academies Press, 1978: Chapter 1.

Because the vaccine is made in eggs, and because the egg supply is limited, authorities would have just one chance to divert production from the usual influenza vaccine to one that countered the Fort Dix strain.

On March 10, the CDC convened its immunization advisory committee and presented the idea of targeting that fall's vaccine to the swine flu. There was some discussion but little debate. One expert described the sentiment in the room as "better to vaccinate without an epidemic than an epidemic without a vaccine."[7] CDC staff later told Sencer "with a pandemic possible and time to do something about it, and lacking the time to disprove it, then *something* would have to be done."[8]

Following the meeting, Sencer put in writing what that something could be: an unprecedented all-out campaign to vaccinate every American. In a nine-page memo to the Department of Health and Human Services dated March 13, Sencer recommended a mass vaccination effort led by the federal government at a cost of $134 million.[9] He wrote, "The magnitude of the challenge suggests that the Department must either be willing to take extraordinary steps or be willing to accept an approach to the problem that cannot succeed."[10]

On March 22, the memo and Sencer's recommendation reached President Gerald Ford. The president and his aides decided the only direction to move was forward. "There was no way to go back on Sencer's memo," one of the aides said later. "If we tried to do that, it would leak. That memo's a gun to our head."[11]

Two days later, on March 24, the White House brought leading scientists together to advise the president on a course of action. It was mainly for show, as there was unanimous support among those in attendance for a national vaccine campaign; those who might have opposed a vaccination campaign were not invited to the meeting. Immediately afterwards, standing with the heroes of the polio fight, Dr. Jonas Salk and Dr. Albert Sabin, President Ford announced a "National Influenza Immunization Program" to vaccinate "every man, woman, and child" in the United States. He explained, "I have been advised that there is a very real possibility that

[7] Schmeck HM. U.S. flu alert set of epidemic virus. *The New York Times.* 20 February 1976.

[8] Neustadt R, Fineberg H. *The Swine Flu Affair: Decision-Making on a Slippery Disease.* Washington, DC: National Academies Press, 1978: Chapter 2.

[9] Neustadt R, Fineberg H. *The Swine Flu Affair: Decision-Making on a Slippery Disease.* Washington, DC: National Academies Press, 1978: Chapter 3.

[10] Neustadt R, Fineberg H. *The Swine Flu Affair: Decision-Making on a Slippery Disease.* Washington, DC: National Academies Press, 1978: Chapter 3.

[11] Neustadt R, Fineberg H. *The Swine Flu Affair: Decision-Making on a Slippery Disease.* Washington, DC: National Academies Press, 1978: Chapter 4.

unless we take effective counteractions, there could be an epidemic of this dangerous disease next fall and winter here in the United States."[12]

Soon after this bold announcement, however, cracks in the plan began to appear. Even while quoting the president's words, reporters noted that scientists inside the CDC did not believe there was a compelling justification to commit to a vaccination campaign. CBS News reported "some doctors and health officials . . . believe that such a massive program is premature and unwise, that there is not enough proof of the need for it. . . . But because President Ford and others are endorsing the program, those who oppose it privately are afraid to say so in public."[13]

Implementation challenges soon exacerbated the situation. After beginning the process of making the new vaccine, pharmaceutical companies threatened to stop production unless the government paid for liability coverage for potential side effects. As Sencer later wrote, "instead of boxes of bottled vaccine, the vaccine manufacturers delivered an ultimatum— that the federal government indemnify them against claims of adverse reactions as a requirement for release of the vaccines."[14] Congress and the administration then bickered publicly for months over details of legislation to extend liability protections, a back and forth that did little to inspire public confidence. Congress eventually passed liability protections in August, just weeks before the vaccine was to be made available.

Another mistake: Trials were designed to test the effectiveness of one dose of vaccine. As a result, the research did not assess whether children, with less mature immune systems, might require two doses. The initial review of the trial results "implied that immunizations should begin by leaving out all persons under 18, perhaps all those under 24."[15] Eventually, officials decided that children should receive two doses of one of the formulations of the vaccine, which unfortunately had been made in relatively small quantities. The result was what one local health leader called a vaccine protocol "so complex . . . in a mass immunization program designed for millions within 8 weeks."[16]

---

[12] Neustadt R, Fineberg H. *The Swine Flu Affair: Decision-Making on a Slippery Disease.* Washington, DC: National Academies Press, 1978: Chapter 4.

[13] Neustadt R, Fineberg H. *The Swine Flu Affair: Decision-Making on a Slippery Disease.* Washington, DC: National Academies Press, 1978: Chapter 4.

[14] Sencer D, Millar J. Reflections on the 1976 swine flu vaccination program. *Emerging Infectious Diseases.* 2006;12(1):23–28.

[15] Neustadt R, Fineberg H. *The Swine Flu Affair: Decision-Making on a Slippery Disease.* Washington, DC: National Academies Press, 1978: Chapter 6.

[16] Imperato P. Reflections on New York City's 1947 smallpox vaccination program and its 1976 swine influenza immunization program. *Journal of Community Health.* 2015;40(3):581–596.

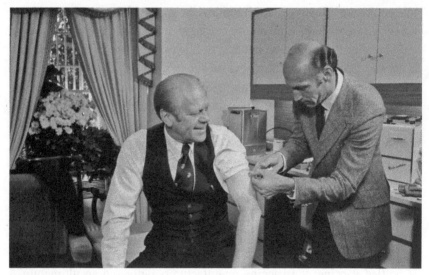

FIGURE 4.1 President Gerald Ford receives a flu shot in 1976

Courtesy Gerald R. Ford Presidential Library and Museum
https://www.fordlibrarymuseum.gov/avproj/swineflu.asp

Vaccinations began on October 1, 1976. On October 11, Pittsburgh television reported several deaths of individuals over 70 soon after vaccination. One newspaper headline read, "The Scene at the Death Clinic."[17] Several state health departments immediately suspended their immunization programs, and the CDC was consumed with the need to explain that the deaths were incidental and not connected to vaccination. To redirect public attention, the White House orchestrated the televised vaccination of the president (Figure 4.1).

Nonetheless, many state and local health officials refused to participate in the vaccination campaign, pointing out that there had not been a single case of the feared strain of influenza since the first report back in February. Even in New York City, where authorities did offer the vaccine, one survey found that only about 16.1% of the intended population had been vaccinated, and nearly as many had been advised by their physicians not to receive the vaccine.[18]

On December 14, 1976, the CDC announced that there was evidence of a possible association of vaccination against the swine flu with neurological complication known as Guillain Barre disease, which can cause paralysis and death.[19] At least 90 cases of the rare disorder had been identified

---

[17] Imperato P. Reflections on New York City's 1947 smallpox vaccination program and its 1976 swine influenza immunization program. *Journal of Community Health*. 2015;40(3):581–596.
[18] Imperato P. Reflections on New York City's 1947 smallpox vaccination program and its 1976 swine influenza immunization program. *Journal of Community Health*. 2015;40(3):581–596.
[19] CDC. *MMWR*. 1976;25(50):1–2.

across 14 states. Two days later, the federal government suspended the campaign to study this potential risk in greater detail. Vaccination against the Fort Dix strain of swine flu would never be restarted. In the final tally, 40 million Americans had been immunized, less than 20% of the original goal.

Within five days, Harry Schwartz of *The New York Times* wrote that the swine flu "fiasco" had its origins in "the self-interest of Government health bureaucracy which saw in the swine flu threat the ideal chance to impress the nation with the capabilities of saving money and lives by preventing disease."[20] Yet what had resulted was the polar opposite of the acclaim showered upon the FDA after the Elixir Sulfanilamide and thalidomide crises. Within two months, Sencer had been replaced as the head of the CDC.

In years and decades since, multiple analysts have dissected what went wrong, focusing on four areas: policy, implementation, communications, and politics.

The major policy error was the fateful decision to commit to a full-scale vaccination campaign so early—and then fail to re-evaluate that decision. It would have been far better, as some argued at the time, to stockpile vaccine and only use it if needed. Yet even as state and local health officials, well-informed consumer advocates, and global health officials pointed out that it was unlikely the disease would resurface, federal officials pressed forward. They rejected stockpiling on the (questionable) grounds that it would be impossible to mobilize a vaccination program quickly in the event of a true pandemic. As Neustadt and Fineberg have written, "Once set on its course, CDC did not establish a basis for review and reconsideration of the situation. As facts evolved, such as the absence of further cases, CDC's pursuit of the original strategy to immunize everyone became more and more controversial and costly in terms of long-term credibility."[21]

Making matters more difficult was a second set of errors related to implementation. Government officials dropped the ball on key logistical issues, including liability protections and pediatric dosing. Confusion between CDC and HHS over who was responsible for key elements of

---

[20] As quoted in Neustadt R, Fineberg H. *The Swine Flu Affair: Decision-Making on a Slippery Disease*. Washington, DC: National Academies Press, 1978: Chapter 9.
[21] Neustadt R, Fineberg H. *The Swine Flu Affair: Decision-Making on a Slippery Disease*. Washington, DC: National Academies Press, 1978: Foreword.

management contributed to these problems. For example, Neustadt and Feinberg reported:

> As early as March 13, Sencer at CDC had called on the director of his Bureau of State Services, Dr. Donald Millar, to head a planning task force. On April 2, at a meeting with state health officials, Sencer introduced Millar as "manager of the prospective 'National Influenza Immunization Program.'" Yet a week later in Washington with funds at hand, Cooper [of HHS] by press release conferred the same title on Dr. Delano Meriweather of the PHS staff.[22]

The federal agencies also failed miserably in their communications. From the moment of the president's announcement, reporters received more information from dissenters than from those running the vaccination campaign. By the late spring, senior reporters on the story had concluded that the vaccination campaign was being driven by political considerations.

The close ties between the vaccination campaign and the White House did little to dispel this perception. President Ford's personal involvement during an election gave the sense that a national vaccination initiative was a fait accompli and that every suggestion for an alternate course would be rejected. Sencer himself later wrote, "In retrospect (and to some observers at the time), the president's highly visible convened meeting and subsequent press conference, which included pictures of his being immunized, were mistakes. These instances seemed to underline the suspicion that the program was politically motivated, rather than a public health response to a possible catastrophe."[23]

Beyond these errors, the swine flu fiasco was also the story of an agency and a leader who wanted to be heroes. It was, in Harry Schwartz's words, "the ideal chance to impress the nation."[24] In May 1976, as the story was unfolding, *Science Magazine* speculated that those "in charge of the war would enjoy an infusion of funds into their agencies and the spotlight of public attention."[25] This spotlight, however, would turn out not to be pleasant.

---

[22] Neustadt R, Fineberg H. *The Swine Flu Affair: Decision-Making on a Slippery Disease.* Washington, DC: National Academies Press, 1978: Chapter 5.

[23] Sencer D, Millar J. Reflections on the 1976 swine flu vaccination program. *Emerging Infectious Diseases.* 2006;12(1):23–28.

[24] Neustadt R, Fineberg H. *The Swine Flu Affair: Decision-Making on a Slippery Disease.* Washington, DC: National Academies Press, 1978: Chapter 9.

[25] Boffey P. Anatomy of a decision: How the nation declared war on swine flu. *Science.* 1976;192(4240):636–641.

Indeed, if the two earlier crises involving the FDA exemplify how preparation and strong crisis management can alter the course of public health history for the better, the swine flu story stands as an example of the opposite. It shows that a vigorous agency response may be necessary to capitalize on a crisis, but it certainly is not sufficient. Strong action does not negate the need for good judgment. Poor agency understanding of a situation—coupled with inflexible management—can lead not to adulation and progress but to humiliation and devastation to a policy agenda.

And the impact of a failed response can last for years. At the end of the *60 Minutes* segment, the husband of a potential vaccine victim looks at Mike Wallace and says:

And I'm mad with my government because they knew the facts, but they didn't release those facts because they—if they had released them, the people wouldn't have taken it. And they can come out tomorrow and tell me there's going to be an epidemic. . . . I will not take another shot that my government tells me to take.[26]

---

[26] CBS. *60 Minutes*. 4 November 1979.

5 | HIV

A S THE SWINE FLU EPISODE began to fade from the headlines, a new public health threat was emerging that would lead to a profound crisis for US public health agencies, particularly the National Institutes of Health (NIH) and the U.S. Food and Drug Administration (FDA). This crisis would raise questions not only about competence of individuals but also about whether the agencies were capable of responding to a grave new threat to the health of the American people.

In June 1981, the Centers for Disease Control and Prevention (CDC) reported on a cluster of cases of severe pneumonia caused by *Pneumocystis*, a rare infection associated with immune deficiency. All five patients were gay men.[1] Soon after, the agency identified multiple cases of Kaposi's Sarcoma, an unusual cancer also associated with immune deficiency.[2] Again, all the patients were gay men. By the end of the year, some researchers had started calling attention to a disorder they called GRID, or gay related immune deficiency.

Doctors soon began to recognize GRID symptoms in heterosexual men, women, and children. By April 1982, the CDC's point person, Dr. James Curran, testified before Congress that tens of thousands of Americans might be affected by the emerging disease.[3] On September 24, the CDC began using the term acquired immune deficiency syndrome, or AIDS.[4]

Rather than leading to a national mobilization against a lethal infectious disease, however, the emergence of AIDS triggered an avalanche of hatred

---

[1] CDC. Pneumocystis Pneumonia—Los Angeles. *MMWR.* 1981;30(21):1–3.
[2] Shilts R. *And the Band Played On.* 1st ed. New York: St. Martin's Press, 1988.
[3] Altman LA. New homosexual disorder worries health officials. *The New York Times.* 11 May 1982.
[4] CDC. Current trends update on acquired immune deficiency syndrome (AIDS)—In United States. *MMWR.* 1982;31(37):507–508.

and stigma against those who were affected. The president of the United States, Ronald Reagan, did not mention AIDS until 1987. Reactionary, homophobic members of Congress and pundits such as William F. Buckley Jr. proposed quarantine, registries, and other repressive measures incompatible with the scientific understanding of viral transmission.[5]

In response, the communities most affected by AIDS began to mobilize and demand essential research, treatment, and supportive services. Founded in March 1987 in the gay and lesbian community of New York City, the AIDS Coalition to Unleash Power, known as ACT UP, became the most forceful and effective voice for change. With the powerful motto of "silence = death" and an inverted pink triangle for a symbol, ACT UP would use confrontational tactics to pressure major institutions in US society—including the church, the media, private industry, and government—to pay attention to AIDS. These included high-profile events involving civil disobedience at the New York Stock Exchange, major pharmaceutical companies—and public health agencies.

From the perspective of ACT UP leaders and other AIDS advocates, failures by federal health agencies were contributing to the deaths of many of their friends and loved ones. Dominic Elliott and Elliott Smith wrote that "[a] defining characteristic of crisis lies in its symbolism."[6] ACT UP protests upended the image of the FDA and the NIH, the nation's largest funder of biomedical research, as defenders of the public's health. The result was a crisis remarkable for its origins in protest by outsiders demanding change.

How agency leaders responded to this crisis would determine the progress against the epidemic—and the course of their own careers.

In 1984, a young physician, Dr. Anthony Fauci, took over the leadership of the National Institute for Allergy and Infectious Disease at the NIH. Much of the research on the strange new immune disease fell under his purview. It was not a straightforward assignment. There were multiple scientific unknowns, requiring the simultaneous understanding of an underlying immunodeficiency and its many complications. Researchers had identified and were beginning to characterize the human immunodeficiency virus as a likely cause of AIDS, and a blood test was developed in 1985. However, meaningful treatments were slow to emerge. The first approved therapy, AZT, reached the market in 1987, but the medication only helped patients temporarily and had serious adverse effects.

[5] Shilts R. *And the Band Played On*. 1st ed. New York: St. Martin's Press, 1988.
[6] Smith D, Elliott D. Exploring the barriers to learning from crisis: Organizational learning and crisis. *Management Learning*. 2007;38(5):519–538.

As activism in the gay and lesbian community began to accelerate in the late 1980s, Dr. Fauci became an early target. ACT UP leaders lambasted Fauci for restrictive study criteria that excluded many patients, for inadequate studies of clinical interventions, for insisting on too high a dose of AZT, and for failing to investigate new treatments for opportunistic infections. As one of ACT UP's founders, Larry Kramer, later said, "I called Dr. Fauci a murderer many times."[7]

Another early target of ACT UP was FDA Commissioner Dr. Frank Young, a former academic researcher who had been the dean of the University of Rochester School of Medicine. In 1987, Young announced a path for greater communication between drug manufacturers and the agency throughout the review process, with the hope of speeding access to needed AIDS therapies.[8] In 1988, the agency permitted AIDS patients to import unapproved drugs for personal use and created a "compassionate use" pathway for patients to access experimental therapies. Commissioner Young even touted the fact that "a computer system has been installed to track new drug applications" as a measure taken in response to AIDS.[9]

These steps did not satisfy ACT UP activists, however, who began to push for more profound changes at the FDA, including the development of flexible criteria to permit faster approval of promising therapies, a ban on placebos from clinical trials so that all participants would receive some treatment, and the inclusion of people from all affected populations in drug studies, including more women, people of color, people who used intravenous drugs, and individuals with hemophilia.

In 1988, Young and others from the FDA sat down with advocates at the agency's headquarters. It did not go well. Mark Harrington, representing ACT UP, later recalled:

> That was a big meeting, where they brought a lot of FDA bureaucrats, listened to our demands, shook their heads, told us they were on our side, but we didn't understand the science. . . . Then they issued a press release about how many common areas we'd agreed on. They had written a press release before the meeting. Anyway, it was a bad faith meeting.[10]

[7] Frontline. The age of AIDS: Interview with Larry Kramer. 30 May 2006. Accessed April 12, 2017, at http://www.pbs.org/wgbh/pages/frontline/aids/interviews/kramer.html.

[8] Boffey P. New initiative to speed AIDS drugs is assailed. *The New York Times.* 5 July 1988.

[9] Gould S. The AIDS consumer movement and the FDA: A potential paradigm shift in health care policy. *Journal of Public Policy and Marketing.* 1989;8:40–52.

[10] Act Up Oral History Project. Interviewee Mark Harrington. New York Gay and Lesbian Experimental Film Festival Inc. 8 March 2003. Accessed May 31, 2017, at http://nrs.harvard.edu/urn-3:FHCL:22795478.

Sue Hyde of the National Gay and Lesbian Task Force told *The New York Times*, "There was a lot of hot air in the room but no balloons went up."[11]

As the 1988 election approached, ACT UP decided to bring every measure of possible pressure on the FDA, drawing on their success with increasingly bold public protests. In July of that year, at the AIDS conference in Montreal, activists had taken over the stage, opened the conference, and occupied the area that had been originally set aside for political luminaries.[12]

With FDA now in its sights, ACT UP sponsored a March on Washington for Lesbian and Gay Rights on October 10, 1988, 26 years to the day that President Kennedy signed the amendments to the Food, Drug, and Cosmetic Act spurred by thalidomide. While this legislative victory had previously been a high-water mark for the FDA, AIDS advocates were concerned that the law's implementation had created unreasonable delays for drug development.

While the march drew a large crowd, it was the next day, October 11, that would go down in the history of the agency (Box 5.1). ACT UP called the action "Seize Control of the FDA." The plan was for protesters to show up at the Parklawn Building, in Rockville, Maryland, home of the agency's massive, boxy headquarters. This was a savvy choice of locale. If Hollywood had to design a massive stage set for a cold, unfeeling government bureaucracy, it would look like the Parklawn Building.

Indeed, preparations by ACT UP included outreach "in advance to the media almost like a Hollywood movie, with a carefully prepared and presented press kit, hundreds of phone calls to members of the press, and activists' appearances scheduled on television and radio talk shows around the country."[13] ACT UP prepared T-shirts and posters reading "we die—they do nothing," with many using the arresting symbol of a bloody handprint.

On the morning of October 11, more than 1,000 protesters swarmed the front of the building. Television cameras were waiting. The news that evening would show activists hanging the FDA commissioner in effigy and chanting "Hey, Hey, FDA, how many people have you killed today?" Activists climbed on top of the building's awning and unfurled a large banner reading "Federal Death Administration" (Figure 5.1).

---

[11] Leary W. FDA pressed to approve more AIDS drugs. *The New York Times*. 11 October 1988.

[12] Beck J. Abrasive activists and bits of new AIDS knowledge. *Chicago Tribune*. 25 June 1990.

[13] Crimp D. Before Occupy: How AIDS activists seized control of the FDA in 1988. *The Atlantic*. 6 December 2011.

BOX 5.1 SEIZE CONTROL OF THE FDA

by Mark Harrington

ACT UP's first national demonstration, "Seize Control of the FDA," on October 11, 1988, kicked off an epic campaign to transform the drug testing system in the United States, a campaign that produced results far beyond its wildest dreams. AIDS activists forced the FDA, the NIH, and drug companies to speed up research, broaden access, provide new treatments which prolonged the lives of people with AIDS and prevented many opportunistic diseases.

It began on Friday, October 7, 1988, when hundreds of ACT UP members took buses down to Washington, D.C., to see the Names Project Quilt. Covering the entire Ellipse on the Mall, the portable cemetery commemorated the names of 8,288 people who had died of AIDS, a quarter of the national total to date. All day long, speakers read aloud from the litany of names. People walked along canvas strips lining each block of six panels.

On October 11, 1988, ACT UP members from around the country made their way to the blocklike FDA building. Perhaps 1,500 activists surrounded the building. Groups from each city, and affinity groups from ACT UP/New York, clustered together in the street by the front entrance, before a double row of county cops. Each group had its own visual signature, signs, and themes; 176 activists were arrested.

The TV news coverage that evening was comprehensive and sympathetic. We were on all local stations, ABC, NBC, CBS, Fox, and CNN. Press coverage of the FDA demonstration was overwhelming. We made the front page in Boston, Baltimore, Dallas, Houston, Orlando, and Miami and were well-covered in Atlanta, Buffalo, Chicago, Detroit, Los Angeles, Memphis, New York, Philadelphia, San Francisco, St. Louis, Tampa, Tucson, and Washington, D.C. *USA Today* ran a story on the front page of its third section. The tone of the coverage was favorable. AIDS activism had gone national.

Among community newspapers, the coverage was euphoric. A turning point in the AIDS epidemic had been reached. In fighting for the rights of people with AIDS, some said, we were at the vanguard of a larger movement for patients' rights, a movement to revolutionize medical research for all diseases. As Robert Massa put it in New York's *Village Voice*,

These activists seek nothing less than a revolution in medical research. They are challenging long-standing assumptions about drug development. For the demonstrators who gathered in Washington, what the researchers call good science is murder—especially in this epidemic, when experimental drugs may be a patient's last hope. ACT UP's critique rests on a single sentence that became a slogan of the FDA action: "A Drug Trial Is Health Care Too."[1]

(continued)

Kiki Mason, writing in the *New York Native*, was even more euphoric:

In 18 months, ACT UP and similar militant organizations across the country have turned the tide of AIDS activism and forever changed the traditional gay movement. . . .

If militant organizations maintain their pressure on the FDA, the process will move faster, and lives will be saved . . .

In the long war on AIDS this past weekend may be remembered as Gettysburg. We still have much heartache and bloodshed ahead of us. We can take it. The tide has turned. Victory will be ours.[2]

A full perspective, "In Depth: AIDS Activists and the FDA," by Mark Harrington is included in Appendix 1. In this essay, Mr. Harrington provides rich detail about the interactions between activists and the NIH and the FDA, and how the HIV crisis led to significant progress in the regulation of pharmaceuticals.

[1] Massa, R. Acting up at the FDA: What AIDS activists want. *Village Voice*. 18 October 1988: 1.

[2] Mason, K. FDA: The demo of the year: With the troops in Washington. *New York Native*. 24 October 1988: 13–17.

The siege went on for hours. Cameras captured the shocked faces of hundreds of FDA scientists looking down from inside the building, the arrival of the police in riot gear and surgical gloves, and the arrest of 176 demonstrators. Mark Harrington recalled that there was "something about the FDA demo" that was "very powerful . . . about people with the disease, surrounding a building that's a bureaucracy—that's slowing down, that's throttling us with red tape."[14]

By the time the protest ended, the heroic image of the FDA was in tatters.

Much less known is that, on that same day, a smaller number of ACT UP protesters turned up at NIH. However, Fauci took a different approach than FDA officials. "I looked at them," he later recalled, "and I saw people who were in pain. I didn't see people who were threatening me, I saw

---

[14] ACT UP Oral History Project. Interviewee Mark Harrington. New York Gay and Lesbian Experimental Film Festival Inc. 8 March 2003. Accessed May 31, 2017, at http://nrs.harvard.edu/urn-3:FHCL:22795478.

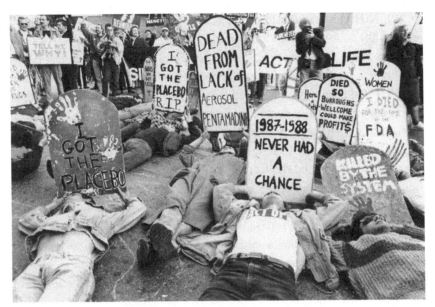

FIGURE 5.1 ACT UP protests at the FDA in 1988
Credit: © Peter Ansin Courtesy of Mikki Ansin

people who were in pain. And that's exactly what I saw, and I was very moved by the pain. *Boy, they must really be hurting for them to do this.* And I think I conveyed that to them, and they saw that that's how I was feeling toward them."[15]

Fauci stopped the police from arresting the protesters and met with several of the leaders in his office. He recalled:

> That began a relationship over many years that allowed me to walk amongst them. . . . It was really interesting; they let me into their camp. . . . I went to San Francisco, to the Castro District, and I discussed the problems they were having, the degree of suffering that was going on in the community, the need for them to get involved in clinical trials, since there were no other possibilities for them to get access to drugs. And I earned their confidence.[16]

[15] Unger D. "I Saw People Who Were in Pain." *Holy Cross Magazine*. Summer 2002. Accessed April 20, 2017, at https://www.holycross.edu/departments/publicaffairs/hcm/summer02/features/fauci.html.

[16] Unger D. "I saw people who were in pain." *Holy Cross Magazine*. Summer 2002. Accessed April 20, 2017, at https://www.holycross.edu/departments/publicaffairs/hcm/summer02/features/fauci.html.

The NIH was moving to turn crisis to opportunity. In 1989, working with AIDS advocates, Fauci endorsed the idea of a parallel track of drug development—in which people who were not eligible for studies could nonetheless receive treatment with experimental medicines. In May 1990, ACT UP led a new protest called "Storm the NIH" involving more than 1,000 people, with key demands including more diverse representation in clinical trials. The agency responded by agreeing with the premise of the protest and calling on Congress to appropriate more funds.[17] That same year, Fauci established the Community Constituency Group, an advisory body that included advocates, and charged the group with a meaningful role in assuring appropriate designs for study protocols. Soon after, with his support, patients with AIDS were participating in research committees across the country. Fauci would go on to oversee studies that identified multiple revolutionary treatments and support projects that would save the lives of millions of people with HIV and AIDS around the world. As of 2018, he is still leading NIH efforts on HIV and AIDS.

At the FDA, however, Young's tenure fell into a downward spiral. In November 1989, in the wake of the ACT UP protest, as well as a major scandal involving generic drugs, President George H. W. Bush asked Young to resign. *The New York Times* cited "a slow response to AIDS" as a key reason for his departure. Even as the NIH was beginning to turn the corner, the FDA remained stained by the taint of inadequacy. In an April 1990 article, activist Larry Kramer wrote, "Intentionally allowed to die is no longer hyperbole, exaggeration, opinion—it is fact. The systems this government has in operation simply could not move any more slowly."[18]

Then, in 1991, a new commissioner, Dr. David Kessler, took over at the FDA. Kessler had cared for children with AIDS as a pediatrician in the Bronx. Reaching out to advocates across the country and to experts inside the agency, he began to pitch the idea of a "conditional approval" process based on an "earlier-than-ideal point along the drug approval path when an urgently needed drug might reasonably be made available to patients."[19] A medication receiving "conditional approval" would need to be studied further before being granted a regular approval.

---

[17] Jennings VT, Gladwell M. 1,000 rally for more vigorous AIDS effort. *The Washington Post.* 22 May 1990.

[18] Kramer L. A call to riot. *Outweek.* 20 April 1990.

[19] Kessler D. *A Question of Intent: A Great American Battle with A Deadly Agency.* New York: Public Affairs, 2001.

Kessler did not embrace more radical changes to the drug approval process originally demanded by ACT UP and others. By then, however, these demands had receded, as numerous failures of once-promising medications had convinced leading activists of the need for high-quality evidence.

The FDA put conditional approval into practice in 1991 for the antiviral drug DDI. FDA staff proposed an early approval of DDI based on an increase in T-cells even without clinical improvement. During a long advisory committee meeting, several academic experts criticized the agency for considering loosening the standards. Kessler and others responded on the merits of the argument, noting the likelihood that T-cell improvement would be linked to better outcomes for patients, and the plans to continue to collect data. A bare majority voted to support the innovative pathway.

Conditional approval succeeded in speeding access to HIV treatments later demonstrated to be effective. After multiple HIV drugs were approved rapidly, Mark Harrington of ACT UP called Kessler "the much more competent and intelligent and reformist commissioner." Scientific advances would soon revolutionize the care of patients with HIV—allowing the once inevitably lethal infection to become a chronic disease.

Essential to the FDA's redemption was the recognition by Kessler that the ACT UP protests had caused as much of a crisis for the agency as anything in its storied past. This was not a case of a dangerous therapy, such as the Elixir Sulfanilamide, or an averted disaster, like thalidomide. There was no single glaring error of commission, as with the CDC's pursuit of an ill-fated vaccination campaign against swine flu. Instead, the FDA had failed to adapt in the face of a new lethal disease—and had been called out by a protest that contrasted the agency's failure against its image of itself.

Like Fauci, however, Kessler recognized that it was possible to turn the pressure on his agency into a force for reform. He saw the FDA he inherited as "understaffed, underfunded, and demoralized."[20] And he understood that a strong response to AIDS was an opportunity to turn that story around. In just one change of leadership, the FDA moved from a commissioner who was hung in effigy by ACT UP to one who would win the Public Policy Achievement Award from the American Federation for AIDS Research.

---

[20] Kessler D. *A Question of Intent: A Great American Battle with A Deadly Agency.* New York: Public Affairs, 2001.

Many would learn their own lessons from the AIDS protests. Advocates for a wide range of causes would go on to use similar strategies to attempt to influence health agencies, with varying degrees of success. Where those affected by illness and tragedy have been able to convincingly call into question the very commitment of an agency to its mission, the impact has been profound.

II | Management

THERE'S A NAME FOR the day when crises hit public health agencies: Monday. Also Tuesday, Wednesday, Thursday, Friday, Saturday and Sunday. The point of studying crisis and response is not to entertain others with a few good stories from history, or to shout warnings at the television screen as crises unfold in the news. The goal is to be ready to leap into the fray. Preparation for this challenge requires understanding four core components of crisis management.

Chapter 6 covers the essential step of recognizing and defining a crisis. Chapter 7 provides an overview of how to manage a crisis, whether it is a simple matter of the power going out in a building or an infectious catastrophe ravaging an entire country. Chapter 8 focuses on the twin challenges of communications and politics, and Chapter 9 discusses the opportunities made possible by pivoting from direct crisis management to lasting policy change.

6 | Recognizing a Crisis

L
ATE IN THE AFTERNOON ON April 18, 2007, a lawyer from the mayor's office called me at the Health Department and told me not to worry. A park in South Baltimore where children have played for nearly a century—known as Swann Park—was not likely to be contaminated with arsenic.

"What are you talking about?" I asked.

The lawyer explained: The park was located next to the site of a now defunct chemical plant that had used arsenic in the production process.[1] During unrelated litigation with the company now responsible for the site, 30-year-old documents had surfaced showing that the arsenic level in the soil had once reached as high as 10,000 parts per million. (A usual level might be less than 1 part per million.)

"Don't be alarmed—our technical consultants are confident that there is no longer a problem anymore with arsenic in the park," the lawyer told me. Purely as a precaution, he added, a few soil samples had been sent for testing. The results would be back from the lab in the morning.

"Have a great night!" he said cheerfully, before hanging up.

My evening, however, was just beginning. I dialed the 24-hour hotline at the Centers for Disease Control and Prevention (CDC) and asked for the on-call expert for environmental health. When she called back, I told her everything I had just learned.

She barely paused before responding. "The results tomorrow will show high levels of arsenic," she said.

"How do you know?" I asked.

"Arsenic never goes anywhere."

---

[1] One of the buildings at the production site was called the Arsenic Shed.

I next called the cell phone of Professor Thomas Burke at the Johns Hopkins Bloomberg School of Public Health. Tom had served as a leading environmental official in New Jersey in the 1980s and was always an accessible source of knowledge and good judgment. I intended to ask him some technical questions.

As soon as I heard his voice, however, I broke down. "How in the world could the law department have not told me about this earlier? How is it even possible that the health commissioner is the last one to know?"

I anticipated that the shocking news of significant arsenic contamination in a local park would lead to public outrage and distract me from everything else I had to do that week.

"Stop whining," Tom interrupted. "You're a lucky guy. You've figured out there's a crisis coming, with at least 12 hours to prepare."

With his guidance, working into the early morning, I arranged for a commitment from the CDC to send a team to Baltimore to study the health risks, prepared a press release to close the park, and developed materials for answering questions from the public and media.

The next morning, when the tests came back showing astronomically high levels of arsenic in the soil of Swann Park, the city lawyers were shocked. But the public health team was ready. I went on local news to announce that the Health Department was closing the park as a precautionary measure while we figured out what had happened, what the risks were, and what should be done to protect the community (Figure 6.1).[2] We quickly convened a task force to review the history and make recommendations for preventing another experience with lost test results.[3] We eventually received payment from the company to cover the remediation of Swann Park, plus new athletic fields and lights for the community.[4]

Swann Park taught me a key lesson: The first order of business in crisis management is figuring out that there is a crisis.[5] Crisis experts emphasize the critical role of this step, with Steven Fink describing the "prodromal" phase of crisis and Ian Mitroff calling the first key task of crisis management "signal detection."[6] Once a brewing crisis is recognized, health

[2] Pelton T. Arsenic forces closing of park; tests show high levels of arsenic. *The Baltimore Sun.* 20 April 2007.

[3] Swann Park Task Force. Arsenic in Swann Park and the Kepone Task Force of 1976. 10 July 2007. Accessed June 2, 2017, at http://msa.maryland.gov/megafile/msa/speccol/sc5300/sc5339/000113/004000/004319/unrestricted/20071157e-002.pdf.

[4] Anderson J. Baltimore reopening Swann Park, closed 3 years for park cleanup. *The Baltimore Sun.* 10 May 2010.

[5] Hermann CF. *Crisis in Foreign Policy: A Simulation Analysis.* Princeton, NJ: Center of International Studies, Princeton University, 1969.

[6] Coombs WT. *Ongoing Crisis Communication: Planning, Managing and Responding.* 3rd ed. Los Angeles: SAGE, 2012.

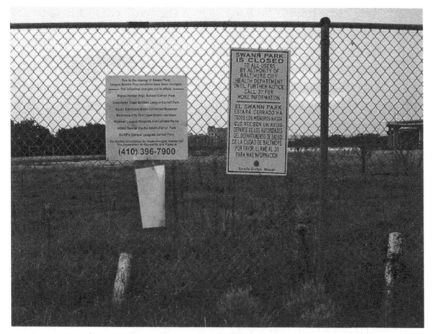

FIGURE 6.1 Swann Park was closed to the public due to high levels of arsenic in the soil

Courtesy Fred Scharman

officials can organize a coherent response, limit its impact, and even make an early pivot to achieve long-lasting change.

Unfortunately, spotting a crisis early is far easier said than done. It's the rare crisis, like Swann Park, that announces itself with a phone call 12 hours in advance. Most crises go undetected even as clues emerge, lost in the stream of the daily activity of an agency.

Failure to Recognize Crises

Why do people and organizations fail to recognize crises? Let us consider the ways.

Bias toward the Usual

There is a natural tendency to place new developments into an existing and comfortable pattern. "It turns out that humans have developed a surprising ability to explain aberrations in such a way that they conform to their established way of thinking," wrote Arjen Boin and his colleagues. "Most people have great trouble thinking 'out of the box,' yet this is precisely what is needed to detect impending crises."[7]

A classic example of this mistake is the crisis at Three Mile Island, the nuclear reactor in New York that partially melted down in 1979 and nearly caused a major public health catastrophe. The events started when a valve that provided water to remove heat from the reactor core became stuck in the open position. When initial signs suggested a loss of coolant, the plant workers came up with many innocent explanations—and wound up taking actions that reduced the water level even further.[8] As Mark Stein from the University of Reading later noted:

> In essence, these explanations enabled them to conclude that the potentially frightening radiation, temperature, and pressure readings did not represent real measures, but were the results of "[measuring] instrument malfunction." This idea was firmly held onto for over two days, despite the varied types of readings they took confirming that something was seriously wrong, and despite information that those in charge had about potentially catastrophic failure of valves at US nuclear power stations.[9]

At one point, an operator at Three Mile Island noticed a massive spike in air pressure, some 33 hours after the disaster had begun. "Dismissed as either 'a valve slamming under high pressure' or the result of [measuring] instrument malfunction.' this later turned out to have been a hydrogen explosion, a highly dangerous occurrence in a nuclear power plant."[10] Fortunately, an expert was able to make the correct diagnosis before the plant suffered a complete meltdown.

Cultural Bias

Social attitudes can impede the recognition of emerging crises. In a 2007 paper, Denis Smith and Dominic Elliott told the story of how cultural respect for physicians made it nearly impossible for British authorities to

---

[7] Boin A, Hart P, Stern EJ, Sundelius B. *The Politics of Crisis Management: Public Leadership Under Pressure.* Cambridge, UK: Cambridge University Press, 2005: 20.

[8] U.S. Nuclear Regulatory Commission. Backgrounder on Three-Mile Island Accident. 12 December 2014. Accessed June 2, 2017, at https://www.nrc.gov/reading-rm/doc-collections/fact-sheets/3mile-isle.html.

[9] Stein M. The critical period of disasters: Insights from sense-making and psychoanalytic theory. *Human Relations.* 2004;57(10):1243–1261.

[10] Smith D, Elliott D. Exploring the barriers to learning from crisis: Organizational learning and crisis. *Management Learning.* 2007;38(5):519–538.

recognize a dangerous physician in their midst—for years. The physician was Dr. David Shipman, who turned out to be a serial killer of more than 200 patients. As evidence of his deadly activities mounted, Shipman was protected "by the status of doctors within society."[11] Smith and Elliott noted "such was the high level of trust vested in Shipman that those with suspicions felt unable to report their concerns." Even after a fellow physician did call attention to the extraordinary number of deaths among patients in his care, the police investigation "was hindered by the view of the investigators that Shipman was a caring and professional [doctor]."[12]

Poor Information Flow

Inadequate communication within organizations can prevent timely understanding of major threats. As crisis experts have noted, "many of the clues needed to detect a crisis in the making are usually available somewhere within the organizations that are responsible for preventing the disasters they encounter."[13] Unfortunately, these clues may arrive in different corners of the agency and never be pulled together into a coherent story.

Indeed, some clues hide in plain sight. In August 2003, the weather agency Météo France released a series of public notices alerting the French nation of high temperatures and an impending heat wave. Yet only after physicians began reporting elevated numbers of deaths among the elderly and emergency departments in hospitals became crowded did the Health Department recognize the evolving crisis. By then it was too late; the heat wave was receding, leaving more than 14,000 dead. Afterwards, despite the public warnings from meteorologists, health department officials blamed a lack of awareness about the heat wave for their failure to take more timely action.[14]

---

[11] Smith D, Elliott D. Exploring the barriers to learning from crisis: Organizational learning and crisis. *Management Learning.* 2007;38(5):519–538.

[12] Smith D, Elliott D. Exploring the barriers to learning from crisis: Organizational learning and crisis. *Management Learning.* 2007;38(5):519–538.

[13] Boin A, Hart P, Stern EJ, Sundelius B. *The Politics of Crisis Management: Public Leadership Under Pressure.* Cambridge, UK: Cambridge University Press, 2005: 21.

[14] Special thanks to my student Erin Feddema for her paper on this topic. Lagadec P. Crisis management in France: Trends, shifts and perspectives. *Journal of Contingencies and Crisis Management.* 2002;10(4):159–172; Lagadec P. Understanding the French 2003 heat wave experience: Beyond the heat, a multi-layered challenge. *Journal of Contingencies and Crisis Management.* 2004;12(4):160–169.

Organizational Myths

Many organizations suffer from the unjustified belief that their own special characteristics protect them from calamities. As Smith and Elliott noted:

> The assumption that catastrophic events are unique and constrained in both space and time can hinder the learning process. A lack of interorganizational learning will result if an event is dismissed as a function of a particular organization's operating systems or culture. This "it couldn't happen here" syndrome prevents managers from picking up cues from events that happen elsewhere.[15]

In 2007, for example, Baltimore City discovered lead in the drinking water of its school system and shut off all the water fountains in city schools.[16] Despite extensive media coverage of the city's problem, other major metropolitan school systems apparently did not seriously consider that they might have a similar vulnerability. A decade later, Newark, New York, Milwaukee, Portland, San Diego, and other cities were distressed by finding lead in school drinking water—and beset by parents furious about the risk to their children.[17] In retrospect, these other localities may have seen Baltimore's problems as not relevant to their own circumstances despite the absence of any good reason for this to be the case.

Normalization of Risk

Agencies can fail to respond quickly to even those crises for which they ostensibly have been preparing. After quantifying the risk of catastrophe, agencies can become so familiar with the threat that a sense of complacency takes hold. "If the risk is small enough, it becomes acceptable," Boin and colleagues noted, "It also becomes neglected, as people tend to forget that risks—however small—can and do materialize."[18]

An example relates to the placement of electrical generators in the basement of hospitals as preparation for catastrophic power failure.

---

[15] Smith D, Elliott D. Exploring the barriers to learning from crisis: Organizational learning and crisis. *Management Learning.* 2007;38(5):519–538.

[16] Neufeld S. All city schools to get water coolers. *The Baltimore Sun.* 9 November 2007.

[17] Dennis B. Facing pressure, more schools scramble to confront dangers of lead in water. *The Washington Post.* 30 April 2017.

[18] Boin A, Hart P, Stern EJ, Sundelius B. *The Politics of Crisis Management: Public Leadership Under Pressure.* Cambridge, UK: Cambridge University Press, 2005: 24.

Multiple facilities have recognized the chance that a flood would both knock out the municipal power supply and inundate the basement, damaging the backup generators. Yet many hospitals have not taken alternative steps to assure safety, leaving them vulnerable to the worst-case scenario. Major calamities have resulted, including at Memorial Medical Center in New Orleans, which had to be evacuated during Hurricane Katrina under dire circumstances.[19]

"Not Our Job"

Perhaps most fundamentally, crises evade early detection because the agency itself has other work to do. Most everyone at a health department has a specific set of responsibilities that does not include worrying about the unusual and unexpected.

As a result, even when staff do recognize signs of an impending crisis, there can be a reluctance to ring an alarm bell. This hesitancy derives in part from having other work to do; in part for fear of being wrong; and in part from fear of being blamed. Crisis experts have written about "the MUM effect," in which "people in organizations have a tendency to withhold negative information completely" especially "if it could make them or their organizational unit look bad."[20] For example, during the swine flu scare of 1976, many CDC scientists had misgivings about the course of action chosen by the agency's director, but in the rush to adopt a policy, they were unwilling to voice concerns at key meetings.[21]

Spotting Signals

Given these many challenges to identifying crises early, health officials and their agencies should pursue a proactive strategy. This strategy should cover three key tasks: spotting signals, pulling in data and assessing the situation, and developing a space and culture to put the pieces of the puzzle together.

An environmental inspector stumbles on a novel chemical threat, or a disease investigator identifies a rapidly growing outbreak. A medical

[19] Fink S. *Five Days at Memorial: Life and Death in a Storm-Ravaged Hospital*. New York: Crown, 2013.

[20] Coombs WT. *Ongoing Crisis Communication: Planning, Managing and Responding*. 3rd ed. Los Angeles: SAGE, 2012: 129.

[21] Neustadt R, Fineberg H. *The Swine Flu Affair: Decision-Making on a Slippery Disease*. Washington, DC: National Academies Press, 1978.

examiner spots an unusual run of deaths, a lab expert has a hunch based on trends in analyzing chemical or bacterial specimens, or a policy analyst reads a new study with immediate local implications. There are dozens of people in a health agency who may notice warning signs of brewing crises that require further evaluation. It is critical that all of them feel comfortable, within the organization's culture, to keep their eyes out for these problems and take action to sound the alarm.

As the Harvard Business School advised business leaders: "To make the most of the many insights available to you, people must feel free to speak their minds—that is, to speak openly about problems they see brewing. If whistle-blowers are routinely punished, or if higher management is dismissive of their warnings, employees will say nothing."[22] Creating an open culture for spotting signals and raising concerns can be challenging. To counter this problem, it helps to keep in mind James Q. Wilson's observation in 1989, "Culture is to an organization what personality is to an individual."[23] Health officials and senior leadership should demonstrate curiosity about potential problems, not defensiveness and denial.

The tone of organizational culture is set in no small part by those health agency staff who interact with external people and organizations. Professor Barry Turner wrote in 1976 about the dangers of "high handed or dismissive responses" to outsiders who raise legitimate issues but who then find themselves "fobbed off with ambiguous or misleading statements, or subjected to public relations exercises."[24] Such actions might reduce immediate pressures but do so at the cost of infuriating the very people who will be involved in placing blame after the fact. Moreover, when the rank and file of an organization see their leaders refusing to engage seriously with potential problems, the clear message is not to rock the boat with concerns about emerging issues.

A better approach is to demand that staff who engage with the media, legislators, and others model concern, curiosity, and engagement. For example, a communications director should look at requests from the news media from the perspective of the reporter. If a series of questions reveals a potentially major storm brewing, she or he should share the signal internally and well in advance of the story's publication.

---

[22] *Crisis Management: Mastering the Skills to Prevent Disasters*. Boston: Harvard Business School Press, 2004.

[23] Wilson, JQ. *Bureaucracy: What Government Agencies Do and Why They Do It*. New York: Basic Books, 1989.

[24] Turner B. The organizational and interorganizational development of disasters. *Administrative Science Quarterly*. 1976;21(3):378–397: 388.

Similarly, the employees who work with an agency's financial and programmatic auditors should recognize that part of their job is assessing how serious the findings are and alerting others to the risk of an adverse report. Most auditing agencies at the local, state, and federal level provide confidential drafts to agencies in advance for comment. Each of these draft audit reports is an opportunity to spot a crisis in the making and to begin to respond. Many auditors will give agencies credit for taking prompt action based on their findings.

Staff who interact regularly with legislators also should keep an ear to the ground for problems that deserve greater attention at the agency. Citizens experiencing all kinds of inconvenience often turn to their elected officials first, and the elected officials often react by passing the question to an agency. Legislators also conduct agency oversight—whether through friendly phone calls or via an escalating series of formal requests for information and documents. Monitoring this stream of communication can help staff flag the beginning of what could become a full-fledged critique—justified or otherwise—of an agency's work.

Beyond these specific roles, agencies should help all agency employees feel comfortable elevating concerns about health and safety. These include holding training sessions, establishing dedicated email addresses, and opening telephone tip lines. Some might ask whether such steps could lead to a flood of reports to be investigated; given the inherent reluctance of most people to revealing concerns, this risk is low. It is more likely that a manageable number of topics will surface for further review and evaluation.

Pulling in Data

If step one is spotting signals, step two is to not panic. An agency cannot launch a full-scale response to every potential crisis. As the saying goes, there are not enough hours in the day. There is also not enough money in the budget, nor are there enough people in the organization. To thread the needle between underreaction and a constant state of anxiety and mobilization, the real step two is to learn more about and assess potential threats.

Crisis experts advise that warning signs should be evaluated on three dimensions: perceived importance, immediacy, and uncertainty.[25] Such a

---

[25] Coombs WT. *Ongoing Crisis Communication: Planning, Managing and Responding.* 3rd ed. Los Angeles: SAGE, 2012: 117.

task should fall to a team led by a designated captain. The team should have the ability to quickly gather data by talking to staff, researching the scientific literature, and, where appropriate, arranging for a more detailed internal investigation. The team's captain should have an ear for danger, an eye for detail, and a brain with superb judgment.

Most of the time, inquiries can be handled through a phone call or an email, targeted to surface the information that allows for rapid triage. In other situations, however, a more thorough examination is needed to protect the public—and the agency.

For example, in 2012, the infectious disease team at the Maryland Department of Health and Mental Hygiene learned of a major outbreak of the hepatitis C virus traced to a single radiology technician. It was alleged that the technician had taken syringes of anesthesia medications for his own use and then returned them for patient care during surgery. A private staffing agency had apparently placed this technician at four Maryland hospitals.

As the Health Department worked through standard procedures to notify patients who might have been infected, word filtered to the department's chief of staff,[26] who began to think about the crisis potential of the incident. He asked a natural question: Did the Board of Physicians, which licenses radiology technicians, know of any warning signs about the technician in question, but fail to prevent his hiring in Maryland? Such a scenario could create a crisis for the Board, which was already beleaguered as the result of a critical audit. Rather than wait to see if a problem surfaced through media and legislative inquiries, he wanted to know first himself.

He asked a Health Department attorney to ask the staffing agency and ask it had ever notified the Board of any concerns. The staffing agency responded by sending several emails showing that it had, in fact, reported concerns to the Board, and the Board had acknowledged their receipt.

At this point, the chief of staff considered acting quickly. He drew up a plan to publicly release these emails, assign responsibility to the Board, and propose a set of solutions for preventing the problem from happening again.

But he decided to wait. After the Board of Physicians vigorously denied ever having received any concerns about the radiology technician, the chief of staff asked the Health Department's inspector general—an internal auditor—to investigate what the Board knew and when.

---

[26] The extraordinary Patrick Dooley.

During this investigation, the inspector general noticed that the emails acknowledging the receipt of key information, purportedly sent from the Board of Physicians to the staffing agency, bore a return email address that included "mpb" instead of "mbp" for the Maryland Board of Physicians. Confronted with this information, the company admitted that one of their employees had forged the emails to cast blame onto the Maryland Board of Physicians.

Now the Health Department had the whole story to tell the public. The department released a comprehensive report about the incident, which told the tale of the suspect emails and called for state legislative action to impose regulatory controls on staffing agencies for radiology technicians for the first time.[27] The legislation passed unanimously.[28]

Assembling the Puzzle

In the literature on crisis, Boin and colleagues refer to recognizing a looming crisis as "sensemaking" and call on leaders to address "the absence of mechanisms to facilitate rapid sensemaking within organizations."[29] In the private sector, such processes are occasionally called "issues management," and experts detail different ways that companies can organize themselves to spot problems and respond quickly.[30] Their guidance revolves around a key insight: After surfacing clues and gathering more information, agencies need the space to evaluate the situation in all its complexity and to decide what to do next.

Even when there is a team devoted to evaluating potential signals of crises, there should be an opportunity for senior leadership to discuss the most worrisome information. This can take the shape of a regular meeting of senior, trusted staff—with special rules (such as no devices) to avoid

---

[27] Maryland Department of Health and Mental Hygiene. Public health vulnerability review: Drug diversion, infection risk, and David Kwiatkowski's employment as a healthcare worker in Maryland. March 2013. Accessed June 2, 2017, at http://dhmh.maryland.gov/pdf/Public%20Health%20 Vulnerability%20Review.pdf.

[28] Senate Bill 1057/House Bill 1529 in Maryland General Assembly 2013 Regular Session. This was the first and only time my testimony was interrupted by a committee chair asking just how fast the General Assembly should pass the legislation under consideration.

[29] Boin A, Hart P, Stern EJ, Sundelius B. *The Politics of Crisis Management: Public Leadership Under Pressure*. Cambridge, UK: Cambridge University Press, 2005: 23.

[30] Regester M, Larkin J. *Risk Issues and Crisis Management in Public Relations*. 4th ed. London: Kogan Page, 2008: 44. One of the major types of "issues" in the private sector to be identified early and managed is the threat of unwanted government regulation. Over in the public sector, an "issue" might be unanticipated action by the private sector that subverts health and safety and requires an urgent response.

distractions. It is often difficult to think about the crisis potential of a brewing situation in the hustle and bustle of daily agency management. The sole purpose of a dedicated meeting time for discussion of potential crises should be to discuss the trickiest questions in a broad way, with simultaneous consideration of policy, political, and legal dimensions of a problem.

This is an opportunity for senior staff to ask whether a problem can be handled through the usual course of business, without drawing special attention. One potential reason to stay below the radar is to reduce the possibility of distracting political interference.

Leadership can also reality-test reassurances offered by individuals within the organization—who may be minimizing risks to avoid the stress associated with a major crisis. As Mark Stein has noted, "The capacity to face and tolerate . . . anxiety increases the likelihood that appropriate sense will be made of the situation and that the critical period may be successfully negotiated."[31]

A dedicated meeting allows agency officials to pause and seek external advice, such as from industry leaders or academic experts, about whether the agency is handling an issue appropriately. This is never easy, but seeking input only from people who already agree is not likely to facilitate early identification of crises. It often takes a leader insisting on seeking diverse points of view for staff to see problems in a different light.

Occasionally, discussion will uncover a threat that requires urgent action led by a dedicated crisis response team. When this happens, the agency will have accomplished the nearly impossible—generating out of thin air its own version of the 12-hour advance call. Then, with a priceless head start, the response can begin.

---

[31] Stein M. The critical period of disasters: Insights from sense-making and psychoanalytic theory. *Human Relations*. 2004;57(10):1243–1261.

7 | Crisis Management

I T WAS A SWELTERING DAY during a hot Baltimore summer. Under the strain of everyone's air conditioning demands, the grid faltered. One of the Health Department's buildings lost power, and the 50 or so staff who worked there were trying to find out whether they should go home.

Some of the affected workers decided to call me, the health commissioner, on my cell phone. Others called the office, and a few even contacted City Hall directly. As my chief of staff[1] and I tried to figure out what to do, we realized we had no plan for how to decide about closing one of our buildings, no established mechanism for distributing emergency news, and no way to update our workforce about plans for the next day. Then someone ran in and shouted that refrigerated vaccines in our overheated building needed to be moved immediately.

It took a couple of chaotic hours to get on top of the situation. My chief of staff and I all canceled meetings, scrambled to track down key facts, and ironed out a plan. Eventually, we sent the staff home, set up an information telephone line for updates, and moved the vaccines. But we were embarrassed. A simple power failure had led to dysfunction.

We later met to figure out what had gone wrong.

First, no one had been in charge. The staff were hearing the full spectrum of possible instructions from different people, ranging from "whatever you do, don't go home" to "leave now." The ensuing confusion led to even more phone calls seeking clarification. Even as health commissioner, I did not have ready access to all the necessary information.

Second, the resources to address the problem were scattered across our organization. The human resources office knew who worked in which

---

[1] The fantastic Michelle Spencer.

buildings, the information technology office had all the email addresses, and facilities staff were needed to move the vaccines. None of the managers of these offices had been available when we needed them.

Third, in our confusion, we nearly missed a significant threat to the public health—the loss of our vaccine supply.

We decided that the next time would be different. We made a plan to switch management modes in the case of another power outage—from "normal," governed by the usual organization chart, to "emergency," which would run under a different organizational arrangement called "incident command."

As part of this structure, we would designate a single person to be in charge and act as the "incident commander." Our top choice was the chief of staff, but if she were not available, a deputy commissioner would step in. We would communicate the switch to "emergency mode" by sending an email to the entire Health Department—an email we drafted in advance—or by calling staff through a phone tree.

The incident commander would make all the key decisions, consulting with me and City Hall as needed. She would also be able to deputize others to perform needed tasks, including drafting messages, setting up an information line, moving essential supplies like vaccines, and assessing for other public health risks. Everyone else would be able to keep doing their jobs as usual.

This new approach to power outages worked well—so well, in fact, that I cannot remember any of the other times our buildings lost power (and I'm told it happened from time to time).

A building with lost electrical power is trivial on the scale of public health crises. But the insight from this experience changed my approach to crisis management. I realized that crises often cannot be effectively managed through business as usual. As Boin and Hart have written:

> Unless organizations have been trained to recognize when their available repertoire does not suffice to deal with the crisis at hand, their operational routines will become more salient during crises (which creates a potential for further escalation of the crisis).[2]

Indeed, the ability to switch management gears is one reason why early recognition of a crisis is so important.

---

[2] Boin A, Hart P, Stern EJ, Sundelius B. *The Politics of Crisis Management: Public Leadership Under Pressure*. Cambridge, UK: Cambridge University Press, 2005: 56.

A useful management approach for responding to crises is the incident command system (ICS). Developed in the 1970s to coordinate efforts at the scenes of fires and other disasters, incident command is now the standard management structure recommended for a broad range of disasters by the Federal Emergency Management Agency (FEMA). There are dozens of books and courses that explain incident command in considerable detail, and FEMA offers free training courses online.[3]

Once an agency has developed the ability to activate an incident command or a modified version of incident command, it is worth using it regularly—including to better manage everyday public health challenges. Doing so builds the muscles of an organization in such areas as mobilizing resources, communications, and decision-making under pressure.

Regular use of incident command can mean the difference in a crisis between a staff filled with excitement and confidence and a staff riddled with doubt or even dread.

Overview of the Incident Command System

Incident command differs fundamentally from the usual course of day-to-day management, by following four key principles.

Principle 1: One Person Should Be Present, in Charge, and Empowered to Make Decisions at All Times

On a usual day, the agency director may be traveling and the deputy may be in meetings. It is common for there to be multiple pauses as decisions travel up and down the organizational chart. In a crisis, however, long waits for action can undermine the effectiveness of the response. Moreover, a power vacuum can lead to frustration and internal conflict at the very moment everyone needs to work together.

By contrast, under an incident command approach, "the command function must be clearly established from the beginning of the incident."[4] With someone in charge, and always available to make key decisions, the bulk of the response effort can focus on execution. The concept of a responsible person extends across the incident command management structure.

---

[3] Federal Emergency Management Agency. National Incident Management System. Accessed June 2, 2017, at https://training.fema.gov/nims/.

[4] Federal Emergency Management Agency. ICS: Review materials. May 2008: 3. Accessed June 2, 2017, at https://training.fema.gov/emiweb/is/icsresource/assets/reviewmaterials.pdf.

According to FEMA, everyone involved in an incident command response "has a designated supervisor to whom he or she reports," and the "manager at all levels must be able to control the actions of all personnel under their supervision."[5]

The incident commander, of course, does not have absolute power. A common question about incident command centers on the role of agency or elected leadership. What happens when the health commissioner or mayor, county executive or governor expects to participate in critical decisions? How can his or her role be squared with the job of incident commander?

An incident command structure avoids this problem by establishing a routine in which the incident commander arranges for comprehensive briefings for top officials at key decision points. The leadership can then participate in making important and timely decisions, which the incident commander can then implement.[6]

Principle 2: The Management Structure Should Be Designed Based on the Functions Needed for the Crisis

On a usual day, many different boxes on an agency's organizational chart may touch a given project, including some whose contributions may be minimal. For example, an effort may involve program, fiscal, facilities, and IT staff – as well as communications, legislative affairs, and management. While there may be standard processes and procedures for bringing all of these roles together; these often take time. To respond rapidly during a crisis, it is often helpful to create a special emergency management structure that can prioritize key tasks.

Under incident command, the response structure can be scaled to the challenge. A small problem may require engaging only one person in the whole organization—the incident commander. Larger crises require more elaborate structures, adding other roles as needed in two categories: command staff and general staff (Figure 7.1).

Command staff report directly to the incident commander. These positions include the press officer, who manages communications and

---

[5] Federal Emergency Management Agency. ICS: Review materials. May 2008: 3. Accessed June 2, 2017, at https://training.fema.gov/emiweb/is/icsresource/assets/reviewmaterials.pdf.
[6] In a dysfunctional management system, everyone sits around waiting to hear from the health commissioner or mayor, county executive, or governor to receive instructions. However, because the leadership is not fully engaged with the response, he or she may not have all the key information handy, and poor or delayed decisions can result.

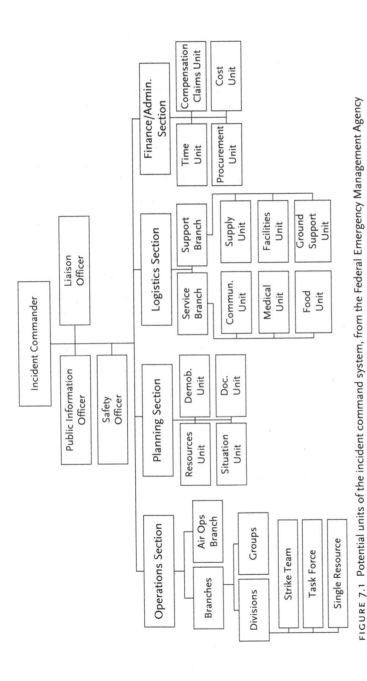

FIGURE 7.1 Potential units of the incident command system, from the Federal Emergency Management Agency

SOURCE: Federal Emergency Management Agency
https://training.fema.gov/is/coursematerials.aspx?code=IS-100.b

coordinates with other communication officials in a Joint Information Center; the safety officer, who has the responsibility of minimizing risks to the responders themselves; and the liaison officer, who handles coordination with other resources and levels of government.

General staff include those working in four sections:

- *Operations*, responsible for "managing all tactical operations at an incident."[7] For example, a crisis response in public health may require the establishment of a vaccine clinic or a mobile unit to test for environmental contamination. An incident commander can create an operation section to oversee such activities.
- *Planning*, which "collects situation and resource status information, evaluates it, and processes the information for use in developing action plans."[8] Crises that last for days and have many moving parts benefit greatly from a planning section devoted to putting together status reports and developing and revising an incident plan that provides coherence and direction to the effort.
- *Logistics*, which provides for such needs as "facilities, transportation, communications, supplies, equipment maintenance and fueling, food services (for responders), medical services (for responders)."[9] An incident commander asks for a logistics section when there are major organizational requirements for a crisis response, such as feeding assembled staff or finding generators to deploy quickly.
- *Finance/Administrative*, which "is responsible for managing all financial aspects of an incident."[10] The administrative section comes in handy later when the bill for a crisis is sent to the federal government for reimbursement.

Each of these key functions is led by a section leader, who can assemble a staff with specific roles and responsibilities, again depending on the scale of the crisis. In addition to these common units, incident command also allows commanders to establish specific goal-oriented teams that may be unique to the incident at hand.

---

[7] Federal Emergency Management Agency. ICS: Review materials. May 2008: 11. Accessed June 2, 2017, at https://training.fema.gov/emiweb/is/icsresource/assets/reviewmaterials.pdf.
[8] Federal Emergency Management Agency. ICS: Review materials. May 2008: 11. Accessed June 2, 2017, at https://training.fema.gov/emiweb/is/icsresource/assets/reviewmaterials.pdf.
[9] Federal Emergency Management Agency. ICS: Review materials. May 2008: 12. Accessed June 2, 2017, at https://training.fema.gov/emiweb/is/icsresource/assets/reviewmaterials.pdf.
[10] Federal Emergency Management Agency. ICS: Review materials. May 2008: 12. Accessed June 2, 2017, at https://training.fema.gov/emiweb/is/icsresource/assets/reviewmaterials.pdf.

Principle 3: The Role Is Separate from the Person

On a usual day, an agency role may be limited to a specific person, regardless of that person's calendar. For example, if only William approves invoices, then invoices will sit in his inbox until William is at his desk.

Not so under incident command, which is designed for specific tasks to be completed when needed. So if the incident commander assigns the job of approving invoices to the leader of the finance/administrative team, then whoever is serving in that role will be ready to help. That may turn out to be William during one shift, Alice during the next shift, and Thomas overnight.

This concept holds across the incident command structure. For example, in a response that involves operations, the head of the operations section may change from time to time, but someone is always the head of the operations section. Indeed, an incident commander with a question for operations can simply say, "Find me the head of the operations section." Some agencies ask their staff to wear fluorescent vests with their incident command titles in huge letters, designed to make identification of their roles that much easier. Passing on the vests at the end of a shift is accompanied by "a briefing that captures all essential functions for continuing safe and effective operations."[11]

Some people in every organization truly hate the concept of separating the role from the person. After all, if I'm the expert in epidemiology, why would I let someone else take over data analysis, even for a moment? But the truth is that organizations cannot be dependent on any one person to function in crisis. Providing training in advance for each role is a critical and essential task of crisis preparation. Once the response has started, empowered staff need to rise to the occasion.

Principle 4: Management by Objective

In the usual course of business, daily agency action is generally guided by custom and habit, based on years of evolution of specific programs and initiatives. In a crisis, however, circumstances can change rapidly, and it helps to develop and revise a written plan with clear objectives.

Under an incident command structure, this task usually falls to the planning section. With input from key experts inside and outside of the agency, the planning section drafts and revises key short- and medium-term objectives, provides status updates based on the latest data, and recommends changes to strategy.

---

[11] Federal Emergency Management Agency. ICS: Review materials. May 2008: 3. Accessed June 2, 2017, at https://training.fema.gov/emiweb/is/icsresource/assets/reviewmaterials.pdf.

After a crisis ends, the planning section can lead a session (called by some a "hot wash") to review what went right and what went wrong in the response and develop an after-action report. Such a cycle of review can reinforce a culture of continuous improvement.

The utility of such a deliberate approach crisis management has been demonstrated time and again, from localized weather events in a single county to disasters affecting a nation's future.

An Example: Ebola in Liberia

In late 2014, President Ellen Johnson Sirleaf and her country of Liberia were experiencing an unprecedented public health catastrophe: an Ebola outbreak in a densely populated urban area. Thousands of people across the country and in the country's capital city of Monrovia were infected with the deadly disease, hospitals were overrun with critically ill patients, and health professionals were risking their own lives to care for the sick without adequate protective equipment. Anarchy was setting in. Although international organizations and other countries were starting to mobilize, it would be weeks or months before substantial aid would arrive and be able to make much of a difference.

Making matters worse, the government's management of the crisis was failing. As Tolbert Nyenswah and his colleagues noted:

> To coordinate the public health response to Ebola, the government of Liberia set up an Ebola Task Force, led by the president. This body was handicapped by its large size, which limited the efficiency of meetings and follow-up, and by inadequate communication with partners and authorities in Liberia's 15 counties. Senior task force officials had competing duties in their ministries and agencies. Members of the legislature were made members of the president's initial task force . . . the initial coordination process was very chaotic and far from that of a health sector response. It was more politically driven and politically focused.[12]

These were meetings "with huge numbers of people, sometimes nearly 100, in the room" with "many people without the right expertise . . . taking up

---

[12] Nyenswah T, Engineer C, Peters D. Leadership in times of crisis: The example of Ebola virus disease in Liberia. *Health Systems & Reform.* 2016;2(3):194–207: 199.

space."[13] Moreover, officials with key areas of responsibility were scattered in "different buildings or locations across town" which "made it hard to have meetings with the appropriate experts present and hindered informal information sharing."[14] The circumstances led to conflict between government officials. Nyenswah and his colleagues wrote, "The bickering was so pronounced that discussions, which should have been monitored and confidential, were circulated in minutes to a wide email chain and media outlets."[15]

President Sirleaf recognized that a major change was needed. With support from US officials, she reached into the Ministry of Health to contact Nyenswah, then the assistant minister of health for preventive services and deputy chief medical officer. She then gave him an extraordinary charge: to establish a structure modeled on incident command for Ebola in Liberia and to serve as the primary incident commander, reporting only to her.

The initial days were chaotic, and global news outlets began publishing stories of governmental confusion and incompetence. *The New York Times* reported in November:

> Even now, three months after donors began pouring resources into Liberia, many confirmed cases still go unreported, countries refuse to change plans to erect field hospitals in the wrong places, families cannot find out whether their relatives in treatment are alive or dead, health workers sent to take temperatures sometimes lack thermometers, and bodies have been cremated because a larger cemetery was not yet open.[16]

Minister Nyenswah began to make changes. He sent word across the government that he was in charge and that involved staff had to be devoted to the Ebola response. Nyenswah then appointed four deputies, one for administrative matters, one for response operations, one for logistics, and a fourth for planning—corresponding to the four major general staff roles in incident command. He established a unit for communications and a unit reporting to him to manage intergovernmental collaboration (Figure 7.2).

---

[13] Nyenswah T. Leadership in times of crisis: A personal reflection from the center of the Ebola epidemic response in Liberia. *Health Systems & Reform.* 2016;2(3):208–212: 209.

[14] Nyenswah T. Leadership in times of crisis: A personal reflection from the center of the Ebola epidemic response in Liberia. *Health Systems & Reform.* 2016;2(3):208–212: 209.

[15] Nyenswah T, Engineer C, Peters D. Leadership in times of crisis: The example of Ebola virus disease in Liberia. *Health Systems & Reform.* 2016;2(3):194–207: 199.

[16] McNeil DG Jr. Ebola response in Liberia is hampered by infighting. *The New York Times.* 19 November 2014.

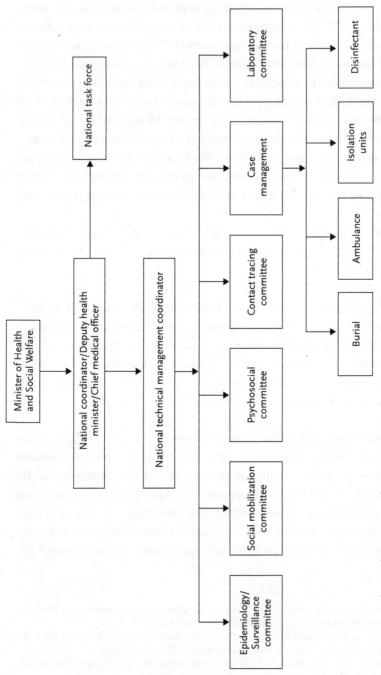

FIGURE 7.2 The incident command system command structure developed for the Liberian Ebola response, from the Centers for Disease Control and Prevention

SOURCE: Centers for Disease Control and Prevention
https://www.cdc.gov/mmwr/preview/mmwrhtml/mm6341a4.htm

Nyenswah organized the response around several critical thematic areas—and set up a goal-oriented team for each. He and his colleagues wrote:

> The thematic areas included surveillance and epidemiology, laboratory diagnosis, case management, contact tracing, case investigation and active case finding, dead body management and safe burials, logistics, county coordination, and social mobilization/psychosocial support.[17]

Each team was led by a Liberian, with support from specific international partners, and had "clear mandates, design features, and . . . common guiding principles."[18] Nyenswah then asked each local area within Liberia to establish its own incident command structure in parallel to the national structure to better manage their local situation.

With his management structure established, Nyenswah focused the agenda of meetings on sharing key information and making important decisions. He limited attendance to key personnel and directed discussion to essential cross-cutting questions. He later recounted:

> There was significant internal debate in each of the thematic areas over issues such as identifying the best approach to make healthcare available; the best approach to dead body management; what was required to provide rapid laboratory support to facilitate sample collection, testing and reporting; how to undertake effective contact tracing; and how these would link to social mobilization efforts."[19]

Critically, Nyenswah used his power under incident command to encourage discussion, not squelch dissent. The process he established led to more coherent decision-making and broader acceptance of the choices made.

Through this process, Nyenswah came to see that community engagement efforts offered the greatest potential for short-term success against Ebola because they fostered the trust needed to encourage people to reduce the spread of the disease. This insight drove the development of key plans, including a major communications effort, known as "Ebola Must

[17] Nyenswah T, Engineer C, Peters D. Leadership in times of crisis: The example of Ebola virus disease in Liberia. *Health Systems & Reform*. 2016;2(3):194–207: 200.
[18] Nyenswah T, Engineer C, Peters D. Leadership in times of crisis: The example of Ebola virus disease in Liberia. *Health Systems & Reform*. 2016;2(3): 194–207: 200.
[19] Nyenswah T, Engineer C, Peters D. Leadership in times of crisis: The example of Ebola virus disease in Liberia. *Health Systems & Reform*. 2016;2(3):194–207: 201.

Go." The messaging strategy provided specific actions every individual, family, and community could take to protect themselves and others. In addition, teams reporting through the incident command structure trained thousands of community health volunteers to deliver key the messages around the country. Nyenswah and President Sirleaf convened the nation's traditional leaders to make a special appeal for assistance, and the traditional leaders agreed to help. Nyenswah gave them each special mobile phones to be used to alert the health ministry of new cases.

Nyenswah may have been the incident commander, but he knew his power came from his appointment by President Sirleaf. He also knew he needed her ongoing support to help the country take key steps forward. So he briefed her directly and presented updates regularly to a small advisory body she established that consisted of senior domestic and global officials. In doing so, he preserved the integrity of the incident command structure for carrying out key strategies and directives.

Faster than anyone anticipated, Liberia began to see results. Burial practices began changing around the country, which reduced the risk of Ebola's spread, and ill patients increasingly isolated themselves at home. By December 2014, only about five cases were reported each day in Monrovia. The epidemic shifted well in advance of the establishment of large new hospitals and clinics; many that were planned were never needed.[20] Three months earlier, the CDC had projected that absent additional action, there would be hundreds of thousands of Ebola cases in Liberia; the final tally for the outbreak was 10,678 cases and 4,810 deaths as of April 2016.[21] Nyenswah and his colleagues noted, "Despite having a later start to the epidemic and more cases than Guinea or Sierra Leone, Liberia was the first to be declared Ebola-Free."[22] Eventually, Nyenswah told President Sirleaf that the incident command structure was no longer needed, and she returned oversight back to agencies for usual operations.

For his part, Minister Nyenswah was appropriately recognized as a hero. In 2016, he received the $100,000 Emerging Leader Award from the Johns Hopkins Bloomberg School of Public Health, recognized alongside

---

[20] Centers for Disease Control and Prevention. 2014 Ebola outbreak in West Africa—Case counts. 13 April 2016. Accessed June 2, 2017, at https://www.cdc.gov/vhf/ebola/outbreaks/2014-west-africa/case-counts.html.
[21] Meltzer MI, Atkins CY, Santibanez S, Knust B, Petersen BW, Ervin ED, Nichol ST, Damon IK, Washington ML, Centers for Disease Control and Prevention. Estimating the future number of cases in the Ebola epidemic—Liberia and Sierra Leone, 2014–2015. *MMWR Suppl.* 2014 Sep 26;63(3):1–14.
[22] Nyenswah T, Engineer C, Peters D. Leadership in times of crisis: The example of Ebola virus disease in Liberia. *Health Systems & Reform.* 2016;2(3):194–207: 202.

Bono and World Health Organization director Margaret Chan, for his contributions to global health.

Other Uses of Incident Command

From a power outage in a single building in Baltimore to controlling the Ebola virus in Liberia—now that's a flexible management structure. It is no surprise, then, that a wide range of organizations use incident command and incident command-like structures for a broad range of responses.

A recent survey found that 95% of utility company officials described incident command as "important" or "very important" to their own emergencies responses.[23] As one guide to best practices noted, the "benefits of the system" include that "it's a proven approach having been in existence for nearly 30 years," and "It is suited to large scale electric emergencies due to its scalability, flexibility, and ability to manage large influxes of re-sources."[24] Industry experts are advising utilities to use incident command for problems beyond outages, including sabotage, terrorism, riots, armed intruders, or accidents that threaten our distribution systems."[25]

Incident command is widely used in the IT world, with one company saying that the approach saved their business by permitting a rapid re-sponse to a system outage.[26]

In public health, local and state agencies have used incident command to respond to all sorts of situations. For example, in August 2007, when a horse stable in downtown Baltimore was found to be a fire hazard, the Health Department had to contact more than a dozen owners, find an al-ternative site, arrange transportation, and relocate their horses. This was a story that attracted the attention of every television journalist within

---

[23] Kullmann J. Utilities and the incident command system. Electric Energy Online. March/April 2014. Accessed June 2, 2017, at http://www.electricenergyonline.com/show_article.php?mag=97&article=773.

[24] NEI Electric Power engineering. New Hampshire December 2008 ice storm assessment report. Chapter VII: Best practices for electric utilities. 28 October 2009: VII-2. Accessed June 2, 2017, at https://www.puc.nh.gov/2008IceStorm/Final%20Reports/PUC%20IceStorm%20After%20Action%20Report%2012-03-09.pdf.

[25] Western Energy Institute. ICS: It's not just for outages. *Emergency Preparedness + Response.* 9 December 2014. Accessed May 19, 2017, at http://www.westernenergy.org/news-resources/ics-its-not-just-for-outages/.

[26] Hoff T. Heroku emergency strategy: Incident command system and 8 hour ops rotations for fresh minds. 27 April 2011. Accessed June 2, 2017, at http://highscalability.com/blog/2011/4/27/heroku-emergency-strategy-incident-command-system-and-8-hour.html.

a 50-mile radius. Enter incident command and a safe resolution to the situation.[27]

A few months later, when new vaccine mandates took effect in Maryland, the Baltimore City Health Department recognized a looming crisis in the fact that more than 8,000 children would either receive the needed shots or would be kept out of school. The department used an incident command structure to launch a broad public relations effort, coordinate with the city schools system to track every student, and establish community-based vaccine clinics. Other counties, which didn't use incident command, suffered from news stories of children dragged to court with their parents.[28]

In 2009, Maryland's Medicaid program offered to cover addiction treatment for single adults, but only at programs that met the state's requirements to bill Medicaid for services. Recognizing the urgency of expanding access to care, Baltimore's local addiction authority established an incident command structure to enable as many of the city's treatment providers to bill Medicaid for services. The result was a substantial expansion in access to care, associated with a major decline in the city's overdose rate.[29] Several other counties failed to see a similar increase in resources devoted to treatment.

In 2014, Maryland's Health Department established incident command to monitor hundreds of individuals traveling from countries experiencing Ebola in West Africa. The structure allowed for the rapid creation of a database, the management of staff resources, and the tracking of all expenditures (anticipating federal reimbursement, which eventually came).

At the federal level, the FDA used an incident command structure to rapidly review and authorize diagnostics and therapies at the start of the 2009 H1N1 influenza pandemic.[30] Key teams included one designated to devices (this team approved a methodology to use PCR to diagnose H1N1 infection) and another to medications (this team recommended a dose of anti-flu medication for infants).

---

[27] Brewington K. Arabbers, their horses, reunited. *The Baltimore Sun.* 15 August 2007.

[28] Barakat M. Parents ordered to court for kids' shots. Associated Press. 17 November 2007.

[29] Schwartz RP, Gryczynski J, O'Grady KE, Sharfstein JM, Warren G, Olsen Y, Mitchell SG, Jaffe JH. Opioid agonist treatments and heroin overdose deaths in Baltimore, Maryland, 1995–2009. *American Journal of Public Health.* 2013;103(5):917–922.

[30] Sharfstein, JM. Statement of Joshua M. Sharfstein, M.D. before hearing on the 2009-H1N1 flu virus, Subcommittee on Health, Committee on Energy and Commerce, U.S. House of Representatives. 30

The Assistant Secretary for Preparedness and Response at HHS in the Obama administration, Dr. Nicole Lurie, evangelized the use of incident command and other management activities as part of routine public health practice. For example, she has noted that seasonal influenza, which kills an estimated 36,000 Americans, is an excellent opportunity to mobilize for community vaccinations. She also encouraged the use of "unified command," a modification of incident command in which multiple agencies (each with their own authority and command structure) coordinate their work deliberately, often by operating out of a single location. (Box 7.1)

Atypical uses of incident command may look quite different from classic 24/7 emergency responses. In place of a large command staff, regular situation reports, and frequent management meetings, agencies may involve just a handful of staff who meet once every few days about a longer-term challenge. Yet even under these variable circumstances, the focus and organization made possible by incident command can prove to be of great benefit.

Use of Emergency Powers

In a crisis, public health agencies may consider using special reserve powers to save lives. State and federal statutes set out different requirements for the declaration of different types of emergencies and describe what options are available under each. Emergency powers may permit health agencies to gather information, commandeer resources, direct personnel, waive existing rules, and even impose new ones without the usual administrative processes.

These are not powers to be taken lightly, and some have warned about their overuse.[31] Nonetheless, every incident management program should have a manual outlining the state of the law, and every incident commander should have access to a lawyer to discuss extraordinary options.

April 2009. Accessed January 21, 2018, at https://www.gpo.gov/fdsys/pkg/CHRG-111hhrg72882/pdf/CHRG-111hhrg72882.pdf.

[31] Haffajee R, Parmet WE, Mello MM. What is a public health "emergency"? *The New England Journal of Medicine.* 2014 Sep 11;371(11):986–988.

BOX 7.1 FLINT, MICHIGAN: MORE THAN SAFE WATER

by Nicole Lurie

The outlines of the Flint water crisis are well known, but less appreciated is the federal government's response, which was comprehensively managed through use of incident command and its modification, unified command.

This story starts after it was widely recognized in the winter of 2014 that the water supply of Flint was contaminated with unsafe levels of lead (see Chapter 11 for more about the Flint water crisis itself). President Obama asked his team to support Flint and, because of the public health repercussions, put the Department of Health and Human Services in charge. As the assistant secretary for preparedness and response, I was asked to lead the response.

We recognized that mitigating the effects of lead required more than access to clean water and fixing the pipes (which was, itself, no simple task). It also involved interventions that would support the brain development of all of Flint's children. These included providing medical screening and follow-up, ensuring good nutrition (there was no supermarket in Flint), enhancing early childhood education, and ensuring safe housing. This was also not a job for the federal government alone; state and local governments and the private-sector partners were key.

While the state had organized water delivery from Lansing, the state capitol, we decided to set up an Emergency Operations Center in Flint, as that was where the crisis was. We invited the federal agencies that needed to be involved (including the Environmental Protection Agency, the Federal Emergency Management Agency, the Department of Housing and Urban Development, the U.S. Department of Agriculture, the Centers for Disease Control and Prevention, and the U.S. Department of Education) as well as state and local government counterparts to participate. We worked under a unified command system, which meant each federal agency would make decisions for itself but that we would work together to ensure alignment and unity of effort in meeting our goals and supporting Flint.

The first task was to establish the goals for the overall response.

I named an incident commander who oversaw the day-to-day response. He was supported by the usual elements of an ICS team: a planning team that outlined, with other agency contributions, a plan to accomplish the goals and monitor weekly progress toward them; an operations team, which got the day-to-day operational actions done (e.g., ensuring kids with high lead levels were followed up, ensuring teams doing home water sampling had ways to address residents' health questions and concerns, ensuring water delivery to vulnerable people); a logistics team, who made sure that equipment, vehicles, and personnel were available for everyone else to do their jobs, and an administrative/financing team, that dealt with everything from ensuring local laws were followed to identifying sources of payment for the various interventions.

A Joint Information Center (JIC) proved critical, as rumors and fear were rampant; the JIC team conducted community outreach and became the vehicle through which all parties could inform the public and media and ensure that everyone stuck to the same message and presented a consistent set of facts and advice.

This was a prolonged and, from the perspective of involving multiple agencies, complex response. Yet we were able to accomplish key goals, beyond making safe water available to Flint residents. For example:

- Medicaid expanded to cover most children in Flint, including for behavioral health;
- The nutritional content of school breakfast and lunch improved;
- A novel food stamp program improved access to fruits and vegetables at the local farmers market;
- State and federal programs together expanded early preschool to include almost all children, and
- Public housing programs facilitated lead screening and follow-up.

Following the basic principles of ICS was critical to this success:

1. One person was in charge, present and empowered to make decisions, for the coordinated response. That person reported to me, and I, in turn reported to the HHS Secretary and the White House team managing this for President Obama.
2. The management structure was designed for what was needed for the crisis. Because each federal agency needed budgetary and policy autonomy, we chose a unified command structure, reflecting the need for independent agency actions as well as the recognition that key leaders' decisions were interdependent. ICS is scalable, and some of these agencies, notably FEMA and the State of Michigan, had their own ICS structures that fit within the overall response.
3. The role was separate from the person. This response went on in some form for almost a year. People get tired, or need to return to their day-to-day roles. A series of incident commanders rotated through the emergency operations center, each empowered in their role while they were there but free to do their day-to-day work when they were not.
4. We managed by objective. While the overall goals remained constant, the objectives and plans for achieving them evolved over time. However, the planning section continued to modify the plan and track progress toward it. For example, early on, a focus was on screening kids for lead and ensuring that infants had access to baby formula through the Women, Infants, and Children program. As kids were screened, the focus shifted to follow-up, and the nutrition goals shifted to ensuring healthy school meals. As the community's concern shifted from lead levels to skin rashes, we designed and implemented a plan to figure out what they were from.

The Flint Water Crisis continues to have lasting impacts. But by organizing the response with urgency of a crisis, the incident command approach was able to help Flint transition to recovery.

Leadership in Crisis

In popular understanding, crisis management boils down to one critical decision—that moment of truth separating an ordinary leader from a Churchill. In fact, far more important than any single moment in time is the structure of the response.[32] Effective leaders make sure that responders have clear assignments, sufficient resources, and an opportunity to raise questions and suggest new solutions. A crisis may be the worst time for a cult of personality to arise around a leader; waiting for one person to make every decision can paralyze all the rest.

Nonetheless, there are moments when leaders must make consequential decisions—and without an instruction manual. As Boin and Hart have written:

> This combination of characteristics puts leaders in a difficult spot: everybody is looking to them for direction, yet a crisis makes it very difficult and painful to provide just that. In choosing, leaders have to somehow discount the uncertainties, overcome any anxieties they may feel, control their impulses, and commit the government's resources to a course of action that they can only hope is both effective and appropriate in the political context they are in.[33]

This stress was not lost on Tolbert Nyenswah as he accepted the assignment from President Sirleaf to direct the Ebola response in Liberia. As he later recalled: "It was a tremendous undertaking for my family as they grappled with the magnitude of the situation under my leadership and their fear that I might be exposed directly to [Ebola] at any moment and become infected, thereby putting them at risk for ultimately becoming infected themselves."[34] Nonetheless, he continued: ". . . deep in my soul, I knew that it was a task for which I had been preparing all of my life, from the moment of my birth, when my father had the vision of me becoming a leader for my country."[35]

---

[32] Boin A, Hart P, Stern EJ, Sundelius B. *The Politics of Crisis Management: Public Leadership Under Pressure.* Cambridge, UK: Cambridge University Press, 2005: 43.

[33] Boin A, Hart P, Stern EJ, Sundelius B. *The Politics of Crisis Management: Public Leadership Under Pressure.* Cambridge, UK: Cambridge University Press, 2005: 44.

[34] Nyenswah T. Leadership in times of crisis: A personal reflection from the center of the Ebola epidemic response in Liberia. *Health Systems & Reform.* 2016;2(3):208–212: 208.

[35] Nyenswah T. Leadership in times of crisis: A personal reflection from the center of the Ebola epidemic response in Liberia. *Health Systems & Reform.* 2016;2(3):208–212: 208.

He succeeded by putting a strong management structure into place, creating an environment for both discussion and definitive decision-making, and picking strategies based on the best available evidence. He also maintained an positive attitude in the face of horror and tragedy— inspiring his staff to do the same. The result was strong local and international support for the country's efforts.

Few public health officials will have to face challenges like those that confronted Tolbert Nyenswah. But all can apply the tools of incident command, as well as the thoughtfulness and the resolve that helped him succeed under extraordinary stress.

8 | Communications and Politics

THE REPORT FROM A LOCAL hospital was as heartbreaking as it was urgent. A young woman in Baltimore City—an elementary school teacher's aide—had died of what appeared to be bacterial meningitis. While infectious, she apparently had close contact with as many as 60 prekindergarten and kindergarten students, all of whom now needed to receive antibiotics as a preventive measure as quickly as possible.

The timing was far from optimal. It was the end of the workday at the end of the week, when everyone was looking forward to going home. It was also the very end of December, so the Health Department needed to find all the exposed children when they were on winter break. And it was 2006, so today's social media tools did not exist for us to use. We activated our incident command system, brought together dozens of key staff, and got to work.

One team took charge of providing medications to the exposed children—quickly identifying a pharmacy and planning for deliveries and a free clinic. Another team worked to get the word out. In addition to calling families directly, the Health Department issued a press release that told the story, named the school, and urged all parents of affected children to call a hotline right away.

That evening, the teacher's death and our recommendations were featured on local television channels. The next morning, *The Baltimore Sun*'s headline read, "City Issues Meningitis Warning."[1] Within 48 hours, over a long holiday weekend, the Health Department found and protected every child at risk. A tragedy would not become an outbreak. I wrote a note to

---

[1] Scharper J. City issues meningitis warning: Teacher's aide at city's Lockerman Bundy Elementary School dies. *The Baltimore Sun*. 30 December 2006.

our staff thanking them for their tremendous work, and I went home to celebrate the new year with my family.

Totally unaware of the mistake that I had made.

The next day, I received an angry text message. From my boss. The mayor. How is it possible, he asked, that there was a meningitis case in our city and I was not informed? I was still in my first year on the job, and I had never received a message like this one. Gingerly, I typed back that I had let his press office know about what was happening.

He responded: Do you work for the press office or for me?

The mayor eventually cooled down, but I heard his frustration. Effective management is an essential part of crisis response. But it's not the only one. It's also necessary to communicate effectively, and to all the right people too. Public health leaders who fail at political tasks are not quite up to the job.

An effective communications approach starts with a basic dictum set forth by the Centers for Disease Control and Prevention (CDC): "Be first, be right, be credible." Agencies must establish themselves as vital sources of accurate information to maintain the public's trust. At the same time, public health officials must recognize that communications play out in the context of ideological debates, electoral rivalries, and other political considerations.

Crisis Communications 101

The primary guidebook of effective crisis communications in public health is the called *Crisis and Emergency Risk Communication*, or *CERC* for short. *CERC* is written and updated by the CDC, based on the "writings of classical rhetoricians," "communication theory," "psychological theory," and "lessons learned from the real and often painful world of experience." *CERC* is available free online at www.cdc.gov, and the agency also provides webinars and training opportunities for public health officials.

Six core principles guide the CDC's recommendations on communications:

Be First

The CDC explains: "Crises are time-sensitive. Communicating information quickly is almost always important. For members of the public, the first source of information often becomes the preferred source."[2]

---

[2] Centers for Disease Control and Prevention. *Crisis and Emergency Risk Communication*. Atlanta, GA: Author, 2014: 2.

It's hard to argue with the CDC's top recommendation. In a crisis, there is enormous value in being the initial voice on what's happening, including what is known and what is not. Private-sector communication experts tell their clients: "Nature abhors a vacuum. Any information void will be filled somehow and by someone . . . If the crisis team does not supply the initial crisis information to the media, some other groups will, and they may be ill informed, misinformed, or motivated to harm the organization."[3]

Even without such a dire view of what failure might look like, being first allows an agency to stake a claim to the public's attention. As in the rest of life, making a good first impression is invaluable.

In fact, agencies do not even have to wait for the crisis to start before communicating clearly. If a problem is looming on the horizon, agency leaders should consider breaking the news to the public about what might happen. This is far preferable to having news emerge from people who have been harmed or become upset, which puts the agency on the defensive from the outset.

A key aspect of being first might be called "being present." For leaders, this means reaching out to affected communities, showing up at key events, and demonstrating a personal engagement. According to crisis expert Timothy Coombs, being present also includes, in today's world, "not hid[ing] from the online world." This is especially true if part of the crisis is playing out online. For example, if rumors on Twitter are fueling a crisis, an agency should respond on Twitter. Otherwise, he says, even if there is a press release, "the organization will be criticized for being silent and miss the opportunity to present its interpretation of the crisis."[4]

Unfortunately, with the speed of social media today, being first is not always possible. A tweet or post can scoop a health agency, leading to a barrage of follow-up questions. Recognizing this potential means agencies should have the capability of moving as quickly as possible, to be, at the very least, the first authoritative source of news.

---

[3] Coombs WT. *Ongoing Crisis Communication: Planning, Managing and Responding.* 3rd ed. Los Angeles: SAGE, 2012: 141. Coombs further notes that to the extent that "a crisis indicates a lack of control and by the organization," then "a quick response is a first step in reasserting organizational control and reestablishing organizational credibility" (p.142).

[4] Coombs WT. *Ongoing Crisis Communication: Planning, Managing and Responding.* 3rd ed. Los Angeles: SAGE, 2012: 27.

Be Right

The CDC advises that "[a]ccuracy establishes credibility. Information can include what is known, what is not known, and what is being done to fill in the gaps."[5]

Being right in a crisis is harder than it sounds. It is very tempting, in front of the microphones or on the phone with a reporter, to answer every inquiry authoritatively—regardless of whether the answers have been confirmed. It's also common for health officials, in the fog of crisis, to be mistaken about what is and what is not known.

Public health officials should do their best to stick to the facts. When answers are not available, it's fine to say, "I don't know" and give a sense of when more will be known. As crisis experts in the business community advise, "[I]n their initial public statements, organizations can interject some kind of ambiguity or uncertainty that will enable them to both to communicate with their public and to emphasize the level of uncertainty they are experiencing at the time."[6] (See Box 8.1.)

Be Credible

The CDC advises: "Honesty and truthfulness should not be compromised during crises."[7]

So. Very. True. The writer Hedrick Smith, in his seminal book *Power Game*, called credibility "the most important key to political survival and influence."[8] Another group of crisis experts stated:

> For policy makers who possess it, risky political ventures become possible, and major political storms can be ridden out with relative ease. Without it, even the most basic tasks become difficult and subject to intense scrutiny by the media and other watchdogs.[9]

[5] Centers for Disease Control and Prevention. *Crisis and Emergency Risk Communication*. Atlanta, GA: Author, 2014: 2.
[6] Ulmer RR, Sellnow TL, Seeger MW. *Effective Crisis Communication: Moving from Crisis to Opportunity*. Thousand Oaks, CA: SAGE, 2007: 42–43.
[7] Centers for Disease Control and Prevention. *Crisis and Emergency Risk Communication*. Atlanta, GA: Author, 2014: 2.
[8] Smith H. *The Power Game: How Washington Works*. New York: Random House, 1988: 46.
[9] Boin A, Hart P, Stern EJ, Sundelius B. *The Politics of Crisis Management: Public Leadership Under Pressure*. Cambridge, UK: Cambridge University Press, 2005: 71.

BOX 8.1 BELLEVUE HOSPITAL: LOSING CREDIBILITY

by Grace Mandel

The murder of Dr. Kathryn Hinnant, a 33-year-old pregnant pathologist working at Bellevue Hospital, was headline news in New York City. She had been found beaten and strangled in her office on the 22nd floor of the hospital.

Bellevue Hospital was one of the oldest public hospitals in the United States, and because it was still run by the city, Mayor Edward Koch jumped in to take charge of public communications.

Mayor Koch appeared at a press conference the day after the Hinnant's body was found. He expressed empathy, "Every murder is an outrage, but this is a particularly outrageous and brutal one."[1] He also showed immense respect for the nurses and doctors who worked at Bellevue. He said, "We don't want them looking over their shoulders, we don't want them to waste their energy through fear."[2] He promised quick action, and announced that he had assigned 50 homicide detectives to the investigation. He offered a $30,000 reward for information.

Mayor Koch also emphatically told the media "This building is probably now the safest building in New York City."[1] The New York City Police Commissioner backed up his claim, stating "There's no reason to believe at this time that hospital security is inadequate."

Within hours of the press conference, it became clear that Mayor Koch was wrong. An anonymous guard told news outlets, "There's no question in my mind that we need more manpower, I'm working with a skeleton crew."[1] Several nurses came forward and reported the fear of lax security in the hospital. One nurse was quoted as saying, "We're afraid to go to the bathroom."[3] A housekeeper said, "There ain't nobody there, especially on the weekends. You can holler loud as you want; nobody can hear you."[1]

Two days after the murder, a man without a fixed address confessed to the murder.[3] He had been living in the utility closet on the 22nd floor of the hospital and posing as a doctor with a stolen ID card.[4] Despite the growing evidence, Mayor Koch continued to defend the security. At the memorial service for Dr. Hinnant, he proclaimed, "Security has nothing to do with whether or not this happened."[5]

It soon emerged that security experts and members of the board had recommended that Bellevue Hospital purchase new technology, which would have prevented the use of stolen ID cards.[5] The security recommendations had not been implemented, and, in fact, security personnel had been cut due to budget constraints.[6]

Within three weeks of the murder, and under intense scrutiny, Mayor Koch backtracked on his previous position. He gave an additional $10 million to the city hospitals for the year and restored $20 million of cut funding to the hospital for the next fiscal year.[7] Despite these actions, Mayor Koch lost

(continued)

BOX 8.1 CONTINUED

credibility and damaged the reputation of the hospital. He lost his re-election campaign that year.

---

[1] Terry D. Doctor is beaten to death in her Bellevue office. *The New York Times*. 9 January 1989.

[2] Hamill, D. The chill spreads. *Newsday*. 9 January 1989.

[3] Kandel, B. NYC outraged at slaying; arrest made. *USA Today*. 10 January 1989.

[4] Fake doctor charged in Bellevue murder. *Houston Chronicles*. 10 January 1989.

[5] Scott G. Security experts: it didn't have to happen at Bellevue. *Newsday*. 17 January 1989.

[6] Scott G. Koch ignites ire of Bellevue staff over safety issues. *Newsday*. 19 January 1989.

[7] Scott G. City returns $20 million to hospitals. *Newsday*. 25 January 1989.

Another word for credibility is believability. During moments of crisis, public health agencies should identify one or two knowledgeable and trusted officials to speak consistently to the public and media. Effective communicators should have the subject matter expertise, solid gold reputations, and the ability to speak in simple and clear sentences.

This practice, however, is rarely followed. Common mistakes include sending multiple experts to different audiences, resulting in message proliferation and public confusion. "A classic flaw in this vein is putting technical experts on air without proper training," Boin and his colleagues wrote. "They use technocratic language that many do not understand and that therefore will be wide open to misinterpretation."[10] During the anthrax crisis of 2001, for example, the CDC used more than 80 different spokespeople, each with varying degrees of access to information and understanding of what was happening.[11]

Another common error is providing overly broad assurances that turn out to be untrue. For example, in the Jack-in-the-Box crisis of 1993, when more than 400 people fell ill after eating undercooked hamburgers, the company initially stated that it not heard of the need to cook meat to higher temperatures. A couple weeks later, the CEO had to admit that the local health department had sent information months earlier about a new state standard for cooking meat—one that Jack-in-the-Box did not follow.[12]

---

[10] Boin A, Hart P, Stern EJ, Sundelius B. *The Politics of Crisis Management: Public Leadership Under Pressure*. Cambridge, UK: Cambridge University Press, 2005: 74–75.

[11] Ulmer RR, Sellnow TL, Seeger MW. *Effective Crisis Communication: Moving from Crisis to Opportunity*. Thousand Oaks, CA: SAGE, 2007: 42–43.

[12] Ulmer RR, Sellnow TL, Seeger MW. *Effective Crisis Communication: Moving from Crisis to Opportunity*. Thousand Oaks, CA: SAGE, 2007: 86–87.

Credibility is also at risk when a public agency overpromises and underdelivers. In early 2009, during the H1N1 pandemic influenza crisis, the Department of Health and Human Services (HHS) promised sufficient vaccine for the nation would become available in early October. After production delays pushed availability back several weeks, there was national frustration over vaccine shortages. At the time, one expert in emergency preparedness noted:

> Although it's quite remarkable that we have any vaccine now, that is not appreciated and the focus is on the fact that we don't have as much vaccine as we'd like at this time. . . . There was so much talk about all this vaccine that was going to be available; there was no mention of all vagaries of vaccine manufacturing . . . If they had framed this [as] we'd be very lucky to get a vaccine, then when it came even in small quantities, it would've been a victory and a delight, instead of a shortage.[13]

Credibility is like gas in the tank, and some of it leaks out with every failure to correct misinformation, every overpromise, and every delay in setting the record straight. When the credibility tank is empty, an agency's progress can grind to a halt.

Express Empathy

The CDC notes, "Crises create harm, and the suffering should be acknowledged in words. Addressing what people are feeling and the challenges they face builds trust and support."[14]

Implementing this advice means going beyond answering questions posed by members of the public and responding to why the questions are being asked in the first place.

For example, in the face of a possible pandemic influenza, a reporter or member of the public might ask whether pets are at risk. A public health official might be tempted to respond dismissively, "We're worried about humans here, and pets generally don't get the flu." But a better response would be, "I can understand why you might wonder what else that you love might be at risk from an influenza pandemic. Fortunately, pets are at

---

[13] Ross R. Lawmakers fault H1N1 vaccination strategy. Center for Infectious Disease Research and Policy. 18 November 2009. Accessed June 2, 2017, at http://www.cidrap.umn.edu/news-perspective/2009/11/lawmakers-fault-h1n1-vaccination-strategy.

[14] Centers for Disease Control and Prevention. *Crisis and Emergency Risk Communication*. Atlanta, GA: Author, 2014: 2.

lower risk from the flu, and the actions we take to protect ourselves will protect our pets too."

Even when the premise of the question is wrong, or even offensive, it is almost always possible to express empathy for the questioner. For example, in 2014, during a period of public focus on unaccompanied minors coming to the United States from Central America, rumors began to spread that the children might be bringing deadly infectious diseases along with them. Some might be tempted to accuse people asking about these risks of trying to find reasons to keep the children from reaching this country. But a better response might be, "I understand that there are a lot of fears and rumors about what might happen. But the good news is that one thing we do very well in this country is keep children healthy, and if it turns out these children are sick, we're going to do everything possible to get them better."

Promote Action

The CDC states, "Giving people meaningful things to do calms anxiety, helps restore order, and promotes a restored sense of control."[15]

In a crisis, there is a premium on "news you can use." The media and the public highly value information on specific steps people can take to protect themselves. Which dangerous products might be in the home? What are warning signs to watch out for? Who should call the hotline? In making recommendations, agencies should make clear that advice might always change as facts warrant.

Crises are also opportunities to reinforce educational messages about everyday actions that promote health. For example, in a series of press conferences about the potential threat of Ebola in the fall of 2014, Maryland's health department promoted the idea of influenza vaccination—on the grounds that reducing the burden of influenza would make it easier to identify and care for Ebola patients if any were identified in the state. This advice was widely reported in the media.[16]

---

[15] Centers for Disease Control and Prevention. *Crisis and Emergency Risk Communication*. Atlanta, GA: Author, 2014: 2.
[16] Lange K. Officials: Don't worry; Health workers prepared for Ebola. WBAL News. 17 October 2014. Accessed June 2, 2017, at http://www.wbaltv.com/article/md-officials-don-t-worry-health-workers-prepared-for-ebola/7089837. "The governor also said now is a good time for residents to get a flu shot. He said since flu symptoms are similar to those at the onset of Ebola, people can help by getting the vaccine. 'That might sound trivial and silly,; the governor said, but it 'will eliminate some of the strain on the system.'"

Show Respect

CDC counsels, "Respectful communication is particularly important when people feel vulnerable. Respectful communication promotes cooperation and support."[17]

A cardinal rule of crisis communications is not to belittle anyone for any reason. This concept remains relevant during crises that are not responses to outbreaks of infectious disease or other disasters—even those related to administrative issues or political accusations. For example, if a critical investigative report or audit generates questions about the integrity of agency activities, it is generally ill-advised to go on the offensive by questioning the motives of others. A credible response starts with recognition that it is legitimate for people to raise questions about what is happening in government before proceeding to the substance of the issue at hand.

Transparency

The CDC's six core principles all relate to, but do not specifically address, the concept of transparency. In a crisis, the media and the public are very interested in knowing what is going on and understandably become quite concerned if it appears important facts are not being shared. Public officials often pledge transparency while lacking a good understanding of how to put this concept into practice.

At its core, transparency is a commitment to releasing important and accurate information rapidly and publicly, even if that information is unanticipated, unfortunate, or embarrassing. In this sense, transparency is essential to credibility in crisis.

However, transparency is not the same as full and immediate disclosure of all information. It does not require sharing unproven rumors or providing unfiltered information so quickly that it creates confusion and panic. It is often advisable—and permissible—to take a reasonable amount of time to review the facts and develop a plan for action.

For example, in 2010, U.S. Food and Drug Administration (FDA) officials learned about the imminent publication of a paper finding fragments of an extraneous virus (called porcine circovirus) in one manufacturer's formulation of infant rotavirus vaccine. A policy of total

---

[17] Centers for Disease Control and Prevention. *Crisis and Emergency Risk Communication*. Atlanta, GA: Author, 2014: 2.

openness would have required disclosure of this information immediately, without any set of recommendations or plan.

Instead, the FDA quickly convened an internal discussion of key scientific experts and, based on their guidance, prepared a set of materials and recommendations for the clinical community. Within a few days, the agency issued a news release and made the commissioner available for interviews. The release explained the findings, issued a recommendation to clinicians to stop using the affected vaccine temporarily, and announced a plan to convene a public advisory committee promptly to make the most informed decision for the future.[18] There was no backlash against FDA for taking a few days to decide how to handle the information.

In 2015, National Institutes of Health (NIH) officials were shocked by the discovery of a few vials of the deadly smallpox virus in storage on its campus. The virus was thought to be restricted to the two highest security laboratories in the world—one in Atlanta and the other in Moscow. The CDC immediately briefed administration officials and arranged to fly the vials to a safe place on the CDC campus in Atlanta. Only after the vials were secured, however, did the CDC publicly disclose what had happened.[19] Again, the short delay was recognized as necessary and did not cause problems for the agency. (See Box 8.2.)

Sometimes, during a crisis, it may even make sense to adjust the amount of information made available to the public. In such cases, it can be helpful to be transparent about a new level of transparency.[20] For example, during a hurricane in 2012, reporters were repeatedly calling Maryland's emergency operations center looking for data on the number of associated fatalities. First they reported five fatalities, and then one found out there was a sixth. Every time a reporter happened to call after a fatality had been identified, he or she got a scoop, which eventually led all the reporters to start checking back in every 15 or 30 minutes. Repeated calls and emails asking for fatality updates became distracting. So the Health Department adopted a policy of releasing fatality numbers just twice a day and sharing the information simultaneously to all news media. This approach was appreciated by reporters and did not meaningfully reduce flow of the information available to the public.

---

[18] Harris G. FDA asks pediatricians to stop using a diarrhea vaccine for now. *The New York Times.* 23 March 2010.

[19] Centers for Disease Control and Prevention. CDC media statement on newly discovered smallpox specimens. 8 July 2014. Accessed June 2, 2017, at https://www.cdc.gov/media/releases/2014/s0708-nih.html.

[20] This might be called "meta-transparency."

BOX 8.2 SMALLPOX AT THE NIH

by Edward L. Hunter

It was the July 4th weekend in 2015. To everyone's surprise and alarm, a vial of smallpox was discovered in a cardboard box in an unsecured laboratory on the NIH campus in Bethesda, Maryland.

Surprise: smallpox is the world's only disease to have been eradicated—and by international treaty was allowed only in two highly secure laboratories. Alarm: smallpox is one of the most deadly viruses known to man—feared enough as a weapon of bioterror that enough vaccine is stockpiled by the federal government to vaccinate every American.

With health, strategic, security, and diplomatic considerations, this discovery was certain to generate media and political interest. While teams from the CDC (with regulatory oversight for laboratories that manage highly toxic "select agents" and the only rightful custodian of a smallpox specimen) and the FBI established operational control and moved the specimen to a temporary secure facility, the questions began.

Was it a live specimen that might cause an outbreak? What was it doing there, and how was it missed when the world's labs were swept in the late 1970s? Were there undiscovered specimens elsewhere? What else was in those cardboard boxes? Had other specimens already been removed from the NIH lab? What was the safest way to transport the vials to CDC, where they could be evaluated and potentially disposed of?

Almost immediately came questions regarding who needed to know and who could be trusted with that information. Transparency is a core CDC value, but with a potentially deadly bioterror agent on the move, there were other obvious considerations. Key officials within the administration were involved, with notifications provided to officials including the White House. But outside the closed circle?

Options were debated as transport plans were being made. Each of the following communications plans had strong proponents:

1. An immediate full disclosure and press conference, following the imperative that we not appear to be hiding important information.
2. Selected outreach to key reporters on an "embargoed" basis, partly to provide some measure of insulation against the appearance of not being willing to share information.
3. Notification of state and local health and homeland security officials, responding to the desire for such officials to know about events on federal property that might affect their populations.
4. Key Congressional notifications, including leadership and those with jurisdiction over health and homeland security. Some argued for a wider Congressional notification, including those states and districts through which the smallpox specimen might travel.

(continued)

BOX 8.2 CONTINUED

All options carried the risk of creating a media circus, calling attention to a security situation that had not yet been resolved. Anyone moviegoer could imagine a lineup of cable news trucks surrounding the NIH campus, or a chase scene on the interstate leading to CDC campus, with potential security risks. The wider the circle of involved parties, the greater the risk of a leak.

Ultimately, it was decided that the security risk was greater than the risk of looking less than fully transparent. There was no information the public might act on, as there might be in an outbreak or other health emergency. Policymakers and other stakeholders, it was reasoned, would understand that we chose security over early notification. Contingency plans were developed for the possibility of leaks. Importantly, key stakeholder contact information was collected for outreach over a holiday weekend.

Late that Sunday night, the specimens were transported to the CDC via helicopter and military aircraft. Early Monday, a staged communications plan was executed. Key stakeholders (including elected officials and Congressional committees) were notified first, so that they had a heads-up on breaking news. Reporters were briefed, and a public press conference was held. Widening circles of briefings provided key stakeholders with more detailed information and continued for the following weeks.

Ultimately, despite great interest in the story, there was little complaint about maintaining secrecy. Multiple steps were put in place to evaluate risk in other labs, including a new sweep and inventory of all federal labs. A Congressional oversight hearing examined the full range of issues. The CDC assessed the specimen and found that it was, in fact, live smallpox—and destroyed the specimen under supervision by the World Health Organization.

The experience reinforced several considerations with respect to transparency.

1. Does anyone care? Agencies have been accused of unnecessarily raising public alarm simply to call attention to their own importance. And the public can be fatigued by "crying wolf" syndrome.
2. Who needs to know? Public officials may need to know, but not all crisis situations rise to the level of public interest. An important consideration is that multiple levels of government (and multiple departments at each level) may have relevant jurisdiction and play different roles in a response.
3. Who needs to know first, and what important stakeholders will be upset if they don't know before something is in the news? A useful test is to project forward to a time when information is made public (or leaks out)—who will feel betrayed, and is there a plausible explanation for why they weren't in the loop?
4. Are there risks in going public or doing so prematurely? These can include health risks (e.g., not causing "worried well" patients to unnecessarily flood hospitals) and security risks.

Another example of managing transparency occurred in 2014 during the Ebola crisis in the United States. Public health guidelines required the evaluation, in a hospital, of all patients with fever who had recently visited one of three West African countries. It was likely that nearly all, or all, of such patients would have a totally unrelated reason for having a fever. However, that fact did not stop the news media from breathlessly reporting that local hospitals were evaluating possible Ebola patients.

At first, in Maryland, the Health Department thought these news reports provided an opportunity to provide important public health messages on Ebola. But as the false alarms began to mount, it became clear that the reporting was making people anxious and stressed, both inside the hospitals where patients were being evaluated and in the general public. The department decided to stop commenting altogether about evaluations of patients from West Africa until Ebola cases were confirmed—and encouraged hospitals to adopt the same policy.

The Health Department could have simply implemented the new policy by refusing to answer emails or return calls from reporters seeking comment. Of course, this would have been viewed skeptically by reporters and could have led to allegations of a cover-up. Instead, the Health Department published a news release that led to a front-page story. *The Baltimore Sun* reported:

> Health officials want to put an end to fears that have arisen when local hospitals isolated patients with suspicious symptoms and travel histories, none of whom were found to be carrying Ebola. In some cases, hospitals have announced the isolation of patients, but state health officials are asking them not to comment publicly on such measures going forward.[21]

The *Sun* then quoted health and communications experts agreeing with the Health Department's new policy. "No news is good news," one said. "The way a lot of hospitals and organizations are handling it now, it just seems to be begging for miscommunication." The new policy was adopted successfully.

---

[21] Dance S. Md. to stop providing updates on Ebola investigations, unless cases confirmed. *The Baltimore Sun*. 5 November 2014.

Rumors

The challenge of communications in crisis is intensified by rumors. Since the 1940s, when Gordon Allport and Leo Postman wrote the *Psychology of Rumors*,[22] psychologists have identified characteristics of situations prone to the development of rumors.[23] These include the importance of the situation, the lack of clarity in official statements, the level of associated anxiety, and the rumor's relevance to the individual.[24]

A few years ago, after unknown respiratory disease led to the tragic deaths of several people in a single family in southern Maryland, there was intense media and public interest in understanding the cause. A rumor circulated that the cause could be "bird flu" or even a virus that the world had never before seen. A national news website published a post speculating about what might be responsible for the deaths,[25] which led to a frenzy on Twitter, Facebook, and other online platforms.

What social media takes away, social media can also give back. When the lab tests came back positive for seasonal influenza, the word spread via Twitter, well in advance of formal reporting to the Health Department. A few hours later, shortly after confirmation, the Health Department released a statement and made staff available for interviews and definitively put the rumors to bed.[26]

Fail to address rumors quickly, and they can become difficult to dispel. An agency can find itself in the difficult position of having to prove a negative. Are you sure that the governor was not involved in this controversial decision? Did the health commissioner in fact recuse himself from a decision as promised? Is the medical examiner taking a suspicious amount of time to determine the cause of death? In a crisis, someone on the communications team should be monitoring social media and other channels for emerging rumors and swiftly working to debunk them.

---

[22] Allport GW, Postman L. *The Psychology of Rumor.* New York: Henry Holt, 1947.

[23] The psychology of rumors, 6 reasons why rumors spread. Social Psych Online. 15 September 2015. Accessed June 11, 2017, at http://socialpsychonline.com/2015/09/psychology-why-rumors-spread/.

[24] Zhao L, Yin J, Song Y. An exploration of rumors combating behavior on social media in the context of social crises. *Computers in Human Behavior.* 2016;58:25–36.

[25] Carollo K. Mystery illness kills 3 in Maryland family. *ABC News.* 6 March 2012. Accessed June 11, 2017, at http://abcnews.go.com/blogs/health/2012/03/06/mystery-illness-kills-three-in-maryland-family/.

[26] Associated Press. 3 in family dead, 4th sickened from respiratory illness. 6 March 2012.

Crisis and Ideology

First with critical information to the public? Check. A credible spokesperson? Check. Specific guidance for the public? Check. It's critical for public health leaders to excel in the basics of crisis communications. However, a public health agency can follow the CDC communications playbook to the letter but still fail to navigate the politics of crisis. And what's worse, there is no *CERC* to help public officials figure out which considerations are the most politically potent and how best to address them.

This challenge is particularly acute where ideology is involved. Strongly held beliefs or bias against certain groups may lead some to question the very need for a vigorous public health response. For example, the opioid crisis was seen largely as a matter for law enforcement when the problem was perceived to mainly affect minority groups. The growing recognition of the opioid epidemic as a health crisis has tracked its increasing impact in rural and suburban white communities.[27]

Other examples include the following.

- *HIV/AIDS*

The discovery of HIV at a time of intense homophobia among many in the United States complicated public health efforts to respond to the disease. For years, the Reagan administration provided few resources for research and care, and many ideologically conservative politicians called for quarantine of affected patients and other measures with no basis in science. One particularly vocal and homophobic member of Congress, William Dannemeyer, spread misinformation and fear to justify his extreme proposals. For example, he stated of the HIV virus:

> It's known to have the ability to mutate extensively, and the fear of some of these researchers is that it would mutate to a form where it would be transmitted between humans through the respiratory system. Now please don't misunderstand me; there's no proof today that it is transmissible through the respiratory system—I don't want to alarm somebody here. But the fear is that it could mutate to the point where it does or is able to

---

[27] Yankah EN. When addiction has a white face. *The New York Times*. 6 February 2016.

be transmitted through the respiratory system, and of course that's what happened in the 14th century with the Black Plague.[28]

Overcoming these rumors and their underlying ideology required years of strong advocacy by individuals with HIV as well as sustained pushback from academic experts and public health practitioners. In 1987, advocates created the AIDS Memorial Quilt, which provided a visual representation of the heartbreaking loss of individual human lives and changed public understanding of the epidemic. In 1988, U.S. Surgeon General C. Everett Koop mailed a groundbreaking brochure with facts about HIV transmission to every US household.[29] In 1990, advocates and public health leaders then brought multiple affected groups together to support passage of the landmark Ryan White Act, which provided substantial resources to care for individuals with HIV and AIDS. This law marked a turning point in support for people suffering from HIV and paved the way for far greater understanding and progress.

- *Zika*

The Zika virus interferes with human reproduction and causes major birth defects.[30] A rational public health response would have involved, at a minimum, the distribution factual information about the infection and its causes, along with access to reproductive healthcare including contraception for both men and women in the community.

However, in the current political climate, limiting access to reproductive healthcare for women has remained an ideological priority for social conservatives—and the Zika response suffered collateral damage.

It did not take long for abortion politics to bubble to the surface. Even as predominantly Catholic countries such as Colombia decided to provide avenues for Zika-infected women to terminate their pregnancies, US state legislatures began considering and even passing laws that prevent women from having abortions for reason of a major fetal malformation.

---

[28] Ford Z. Flashback to 1989—Anti-gay Rep. Dannemeyer propagated airborne threat of AIDS. Thinkprogress.org. 6 June 2011. Accessed June 11, 2017, at https://thinkprogress.org/flashback-to-1989-anti-gay-rep-dannemeyer-propagated-airborne-threat-of-aids-c81d8ba8f3c2.

[29] The C. Everett Koop Papers. AIDS, the Surgeon General, and the Politics of Public Health. Profiles in Science. U.S. National Library of Medicine. Accessed June 2, 2017, at https://profiles.nlm.nih.gov/ps/retrieve/Narrative/QQ/p-nid/87.

[30] Sharfstein J. JAMA Forum: The Zika virus and abortion politics. 11 May 2016. Accessed June 2, 2017, at https://newsatjama.jama.com/2016/05/11/jama-forum-the-zika-virus-and-abortion-politics/.

Right alongside the abortion issue was a fight over Planned Parenthood, an organization targeted for zero funding by many in the Republican party. Even as Zika began to spread in the United States in 2016, the Republican-led Congress delayed appropriating funding for the response because some might find its way to Planned Parenthood. These political considerations increased the degree of difficulty facing public health officials and delayed Congressional appropriations for many months.

The logjam was broken for unexpected reasons. In September 2016, a Zika outbreak in Miami Beach led health officials to advise against travel there for women who are or might become pregnant. Florida Senator Marco Rubio—normally a reliable vote for social conservatives—then began push for the release of federal funds. Rubio expressed his concern that Zika is not just a healthcare issue to *The Miami Herald*: "It is hurting small businesses. . . . Miami Beach as a city is going to see tax revenues go down. It's going to hurt one of the engines of our tourism sector."[31]

Public health officials might prefer action be based on health facts rather than economic consequences, but in a crisis, it may be too much to expect support for all the right reasons. It is sometimes necessary to go with what works.

Politicians and Crisis

As the old saying goes, the most dangerous place in the world is between a politician and a camera. During a public health crisis, this means that health officials often need to figure out a way to constructively engage political leaders in communications and management. Navigating these waters in the middle of a crisis can be treacherous.

As seen in Chapter 4, President Ford insisted on having a leading, public role in the swine flu crisis of 1976. His hands-on approach backfired, however, as his strong support for a national vaccination campaign made it difficult for health officials to change course as the facts warranted.

History is filled with truly epic examples of politicians or political leaders mishandling a crisis response. Famously, in 1990, the British politician serving as agriculture minister fed his four-year-old daughter a hamburger on national television in an attempt to demonstrate there was no risk of mad cow disease (Figure 8.1).[32] One reporter described the scene:

---

[31] Wise L. Florida businesses are also a victim of Zika, Sen. Marco Rubio says. *Miami Herald.* 8 September 2016.
[32] Lee A. What became of Cordelia Gummer, the Mad Cow girl? *Sunday Express.* 16 May 2015.

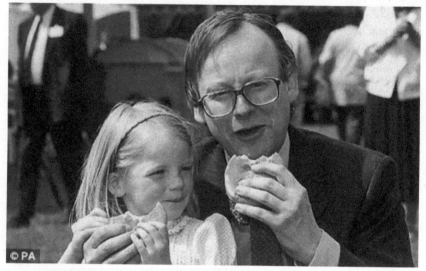

FIGURE 8.1 The British Agricultural Minister and his daughter
SOURCE: PA Images

The little girl takes one hesitant nibble then turns away disdainfully.

"It's absolutely delicious," exclaims her dad taking a bite, but she's having no more of it.[33]

When evidence later demonstrated a genuine risk to British consumers, the result was a historic public relations disaster.

Similarly, in 1991, during a cholera epidemic, the Peruvian prime minister, his wife, and leading government ministers went on national television to eat the national dish of ceviche to demonstrate it was safe.[34] "Within days," *The New York Times* reported, "hospital admissions for cholera soared."[35]

Partisan politics can also undermine the nuts and bolts of crisis response. For example, in late summer of 2014, when CDC Director Dr. Thomas Frieden called attention to the urgent need to direct resources to an outbreak of the Ebola virus in Liberia, Sierra Leone, and Guinea, he explained that strong action overseas would further reduce the minimal risk at home. Yet this message had trouble penetrating in a political environment complicated by deep divisions over the issue of immigration.

---

[33] Lee A. What became of Cordelia Gummer, the Mad Cow girl? *Sunday Express*. 16 May 2015.

[34] Brook J. Cholera kills 1,100 in Peru and marches on, reaching the Brazilian border. *The New York Times*. 19 April 1991.

[35] Brook J. Cholera kills 1,100 in Peru and marches on, reaching the Brazilian border. *The New York Times*. 19 April 1991.

At one hearing, a member of Congress admonished (and astonished) Frieden and other experts by saying, "Every outbreak novel or zombie movie you see starts with somebody from the government sitting in front of a panel like this saying there's nothing to worry about."[36] Against the evidence of what might work to contain the disease, political candidates demanded closing the borders, and governors ordered needless quarantines of healthcare workers.[37] Some commentators accused Republicans in Congress of sowing fear and panic in advance of the midterm elections.[38]

Concern over politicians getting involved and messing up a response is an important reason why some public health officials may be reluctant to treat a problem as a crisis in the first place.[39] Yet trying to manage a major problem below the political radar can be dangerous too, especially when political leaders are needed to counter bias and ideology or can help to mobilize resources unavailable to health agencies (see "Rethinking Science and Politics" in Appendix 2).

Figuring out the best way to engage elected leaders is a core aspect of political judgment. If involvement by politicians is desired (or inevitable), health officials have three ways to guide them to more effective involvement in the response.

Divide and conquer the job of crisis communications. Elected leaders should provide the high-level overviews to the public while leaving the details to health officials. Ideally, this involves a clear explanation that the health response is being managed by the health agency.

Involve external experts. Academic experts, practicing physicians, hospital executives, and others can reassure the public that statements and measures are not part of a hidden political agenda—and also provide a source of good judgment to keep political leaders in check. Indeed, in the case of Ebola, the CDC, state health departments, and other public health agencies worked closely with hospitals, organizations of nurses, and others to provide independent and trustworthy validation of key

---

[36] Chuck Todd: Are Republicans "overdoing" rhetoric on Ebola? RealClearPolitics. 19 October 2014. Accessed May 31, 2017, at http://www.realclearpolitics.com/video/2014/10/19/chuck_todd_are_republicans_overdoing_rhetoric_on_ebola.html.

[37] Nuzzo JB, Cicero AJ, Waldhorn R, Inglesby TV. Travel bans will increase the damage wrought by Ebola. *Biosecurity and Bioterrorism.* 2014 Nov-Dec;12(6):306–309.

[38] Beutler B. Republicans want you to be terrified of Ebola—So you'll vote for them. *The New Republic.* 16 October 2014. Accessed June 2, 2017, at https://newrepublic.com/article/119851/republicans-spread-ebola-paranoia-blame-obama-ahead-midterms.

[39] When a staff person suggests treating a problem is a crisis, one health official told me that she responds, "Be careful what you wish for."

guidance.[40] At especially trying times, health officials can convene an in-dependent committee to provide guidance and, credibility to public health efforts (see Appendix 5: On Fear, Distrust, and Ebola).

Steer clear of political bickering. The strength of a health agency comes from its expertise and dedication, not from sharply worded retorts. Even when tempted, health officials should resist maligning the motives of political figures, even those in the opposition, during a crisis. It is far better to maintain focus on a successful response.

Ultimately, whether a politician boosts or undermines a crisis response depends a great deal on the politician.[41] The more that elected leaders can understand that the best politics come from a successful crisis response, the more likely it is that they will be willing to defer the core communications work to an agency that has credibility with the public.

Crisis and Self-Promotion

How much credit should health officials take publicly for their actions during a crisis? Every official wants to appear strong and responsive, part of an organization that is saving lives under the most difficult of circumstances. It is also important for the public to understand what is being done to address key challenges. However, the image of an effective agency will soon crumble without the facts behind it, and journalists and others can see through false bravado. There is also the chance that a polit-ical leader may be miffed to see public health officials earning too much praise.

Health officials should keep in mind that it is the successful manage-ment of a crisis that provides the greatest long-term rewards. Instead of viewing the media solely as an avenue for receiving and transmitting updates, agencies can create deeper partnerships to inform the public. For example, health officials might allow reporters to join agency staff in the field and report independently on what they see. Or health officials might provide an in-depth briefing on the use of an incident command structure. Testimony before Congress about the FDA's first use of such a

---

[40] Sharfstein JM. On fear, distrust, and Ebola. *Journal of the American Medical Association.* 2015 Feb 24;313(8):784.

[41] I had the tremendous benefit of working for political leaders with great judgment in crisis: Mayor and Governor Martin O'Malley, Mayor Sheila Dixon, HHS Secretary Kathleen Sebelius, and Congressman Henry A. Waxman.

management approach, which occurred during the H1N1 influenza pandemic, was especially well received.[42]

Telling the Story of Crisis

Communications in crisis is about more than facts; it is about putting the facts together in a way to facilitate understanding. Arjen Boin and his colleagues have described this as "meaning making"—or "communicating a persuasive story line (a narrative) that explains what happened, why it had to be that way, what its repercussions are, how it can be resolved, who can be relied upon to do so, and who is to blame."[43]

Meaning making is a useful concept that sheds light on some of the key moments of public health crisis management. FDA officials helped shape powerful narratives in 1938 and 1962, narratives about an agency that fought for the health of the American people and exposed gaps in the law that needed to be fixed. In 1976, by contrast, CDC officials lost control of their narrative, leaving others like *60 Minutes* and, later, anti-vaccine activists, to generate lessons from the swine flu crisis. In a crisis, each public communication contributes, as individual bricks, to the building of meaning. As the next chapter illustrates, success in this effort creates opportunities for previously unimaginable progress and long-lasting policy change.

---

[42] Sharfstein, JM. 2009-H1N1 flu virus. Statement of Joshua M. Sharfstein, M.D., Principal Deputy Commissioner and Acting Commissioner, Food and Drug Administration, Department of Health and Human Service before the Subcommittee on Health, Committee on Energy and Commerce, U.S. House of Representatives. 30 April 2009. Accessed January 21, 2018, at https://www.gpo.gov/fdsys/pkg/CHRG-111hhrg72882/pdf/CHRG-111hhrg72882.pdf.

In this testimony, I told Congress: "As soon as we became aware of the 2009-H1N1 flu virus outbreak, I asked Dr. Jesse Goodman, FDA's Acting Chief Scientist and Deputy Commissioner for Scientific and Medical Programs, to coordinate and lead FDA's efforts on the 2009-H1N1 flu virus. Dr. Goodman previously directed FDA's Center for Biologics Evaluation and Research and is a world-recognized infectious disease expert with extensive experience in issues related to influenza vaccine development and evaluation.

"Dr. Goodman leads an incident management approach that now includes seven substantive teams, which are cross-cutting and include staff from across the FDA as needed. All of FDA's Centers are engaged in this important work.

"These teams work with the Department, CDC, other agencies, national and international partners. The teams include: Vaccine Team, Antiviral Team, In Vitro Diagnostics Team, Personal Protection Team, Blood Team, Shortage Team, and the Consumer Protection Team.

"The incident management structure also includes an operations section, a logistics section, and a communications section that coordinates external relations, including media, stakeholders, international, legislative, and Web site development. It includes FDA senior-level health, international, and legal advisers."

[43] Boin A, Hart P, Stern EJ, Sundelius B. *The Politics of Crisis Management: Public Leadership Under Pressure.* Cambridge, UK: Cambridge University Press, 2005: 69–70.

9 | Preventing the Next Crisis

I N SEPTEMBER 2012, A GRUESOME story hit the news in Maryland. One person died and two were hospitalized with severe "flesh eating" bacterial infections after undergoing liposuction in a clinic called the Monarch Med Spa.[1]

At the time, I was serving as secretary of the Maryland Department of Health and Mental Hygiene. One of the many strengths of the department is its top-notch infectious disease team. This team quickly sprang into action. Working with local health staff, our experts located the facility in a nondescript office park in Timonium, Maryland, and conducted an emergency inspection. It did not take long to find gross neglect of basic procedures of sanitation. Problems included:

> [V]isibly dirty equipment, no separation of clean and dirty areas for equipment sterilization, a clogged sink in the liposuction procedure room with debris and liquid leaking onto surgical supplies stored underneath, open surgical scrub materials, nonsterile surgical dressing stored open in high traffic areas, autoclave logs unavailable, expired supplies on shelves, and unlabeled opened multi-use lidocaine vials.[2]

I quickly signed an order finding that conditions at the Monarch Med Spa facility "endanger the public health" and requiring that "all operations

---

[1] Dance S. Timonium cosmetic surgery center shut down amid investigation into infections, one death. *The Baltimore Sun.* 19 September 2012.
[2] Office of Infectious Disease Epidemiology and Outbreak Response, Maryland Department of Health and Mental Hygiene. Summary Report: Outbreak 2012–2235. September 2013. Accessed June 2, 2017, at http://dhmh.maryland.gov/docs/GAS%20Outbreak%20Final%20Report%200913.pdf.

at the facility should cease until . . . the threat to the public health has abated."[3]

Problem solved? Yes—and no. The immediate danger had passed. But I also recognized that Maryland was just one of many states where "med spas" had harmed patients seeking cosmetic procedures.

USA Today had recently published a major investigation of these clinics across the country, revealing a pattern of poorly trained physicians failing to follow basic standards of care, with devastating results. "*USA Today* reviewed dozens of photos—most too graphic to publish—and cases involving fatalities and patients with horrific scars and infections after cosmetic treatments by doctors who were not board-certified to practice plastic surgery," the newspaper reported. "These include third-degree burns across the backs and stomachs of laser liposuction victims; implants protruding out of massively infected breasts; and lumps and wounds in liposuction patients that look like the result of stabbings."[4]

Yikes. As the cabinet official with responsibility for the health of people in Maryland, I was not interested in just sitting around and waiting for the next screening of this horror show. So even as I was signing the order to shut down the clinic, I asked our team for ideas about what we could do to prevent such a disaster from happening again. The department's chief inspector explained there were no standards or inspections applicable to these clinics other than the simple fact that the doctor required a medical license. That meant Marylanders remained at high risk for the next time a "med spa" operator came into town.

Unless.

Unless we could convince the Maryland General Assembly to give the Health Department authority to require a special license for "medical spas." With a license requirement, the Health Department could regularly inspect these clinics against basic standards of infection control—before the clinics were open for business. We made a plan to seek public comment on possible solutions, including the licensure option, and then propose legislation, if appropriate, in the upcoming legislative session of the Maryland General Assembly due to start in a few months.

---

[3] Monarch Med Spa order to cease operations. Maryland Department of Health and Mental Hygiene. Accessed June 2, 2017, at https://archive.org/stream/435390-monarch-medical-spa-order-to-cease-operations/435390-monarch-medical-spa-order-to-cease-operations_djvu.txt.

[4] O'Donnell J. Lack of training can be deadly in cosmetic surgery. *USA Today.* 15 September 2011.

With public attention focused on the outbreak of "flesh eating" bacteria, there was no time to waste. At the bottom of our news release announcing the order to close down the Monarch Spa, we appended this line: "Cosmetic surgery centers in Maryland are not currently subject to state licensure."[5] Within several weeks, we requested public comment on what could be done. Then, in advance of the legislative session, we worked with reporters to shine a light on the policy failure.

Just before the legislative session began, the local ABC news affiliate aired an extensive investigation of cosmetic surgery clinics in Maryland. The report included interviews with the family of the patient who died, a leading patient safety expert at Johns Hopkins, and me. It began:

> When you dine out, an inspection lets you know the restaurant is safe. The same is true with your car and your daycare. The state looks at all these things to protect you from harm. But sometimes we just assume things are getting a closer look, especially when it comes to health care.[6]

With our help, the report framed the tragedy not just as about an incompetent doctor or a poorly run clinic but about a need for greater oversight. The reporter stated:

> Monarch was forced to close and the [Health Department] release on the case contained a line that stunned the . . . family, stating, "Cosmetic surgery centers in Maryland are not currently subject to state licensure." The loophole shocked the . . . family [of the victim], but Monarch is not the only clinic lacking in oversight. ABC2 investigators found other cosmetic surgery centers across Maryland that could fit into this category. The doctors who work there are licensed, regulated and if need be, punished, by the Maryland Board of Physicians. But the centers where they work are not necessarily overseen.[7]

---

[5] DiMarco N. Monarch Med Spa shut down amid investigation. *Lutherville Patch.* 19 September 2012. Accessed June 2, 2017, at https://patch.com/maryland/timonium/monarch-med-spa-shut-down-amid-investigation.

[6] Sterman J. Family of medspa patient talks for first time to expose medical loophole in Maryland. WMAR. 31 January 2013. Accessed June 2, 2017, at http://www.abc2news.com/news/local-news/investigations/family-of-medspa-patient-talks-for-first-time-to-expose-medical-loophole-in-maryland.

[7] Sterman J. Family of medspa patient talks for first time to expose medical loophole in Maryland. WMAR. 31 January 2013. Accessed June 2, 2017, at http://www.abc2news.com/news/local-news/investigations/family-of-medspa-patient-talks-for-first-time-to-expose-medical-loophole-in-maryland.

I was quoted in the story as saying, "It's a loophole we think we should be closed . . . I don't want to hear about outbreaks where people are dying in the state of Maryland where it could have been prevented."[8]

We then worked with advocates and legislators to support new legislation. Within several weeks, the Maryland General Assembly unanimously passed and the governor signed a bill to establish a new licensing and inspection process for cosmetic surgery clinics.

Would the law have passed without a strategic push from Health Department? Maybe, maybe not. Once the problem faded from the news, legislators might have focused on more pressing problems. Could we have successfully advocated the legislation in the absence of an outbreak? Doubtful. The crisis created the opportunity for change; the response took advantage of that opportunity.

For public health officials, this is the dream: not just to successfully manage a difficult situation but to translate the response into lasting, positive reform that might never have otherwise happened. Like a triple axel jump in figure skating, however, success is beautiful to behold, but failure is not pretty.

There are three parts of this triple axel for public health leaders: establishing credibility with key audiences, providing a coherent explanation of the problem, and proposing specific and realistic solutions. At each stage, there are a number of opportunities to fall flat on the ice.

Establishing Credibility

In a crisis, a strong and well-communicated response establishes the credibility of a public health agency and its leaders. Like dropping coins in a piggy bank, each action and public statement builds up a store of goodwill and understanding.

In the case of the Monarch Med Spa, the Health Department's first action had been to investigate, and its second was to shut down the facility to protect the public. These prompt steps made it clear that the Health Department was in charge and meant business. This head of steam made it possible to pivot quickly to a discussion of long-term solutions.

Move too early to assess the causes of a problem, however, and two risks appear. First, the public may perceive an attempt to dodge responsibility

---

[8] Sterman J. Family of medspa patient talks for first time to expose medical loophole in Maryland. WMAR. 31 January 2013. Accessed June 2, 2017, at http://www.abc2news.com/news/local-news/investigations/family-of-medspa-patient-talks-for-first-time-to-expose-medical-loophole-in-maryland.

and assign blame, rather than to take charge and fulfill the primary responsibility of assuring safety. During the Flint water crisis, for example, the Environmental Protection Agency's (EPA) regional office focused on technicalities about its own jurisdiction and gaps in the underlying rules rather than responded with a clear effort to address the problem.[9] This response infuriated those advocating for the residents of Flint, and the EPA's delay, once recognized, led the agency's regional director to resign.

Second, if there is too much focus on the long-term plan, the agency may become distracted and fail to do what is urgently needed to stabilize the situation. The result may be a hemorrhaging of the credibility required to persuade the public and legislators of the need for reform.

At the same time, it is a poor idea for health agencies to wait until the very, very end of a crisis to discuss policy solutions, because there are also risks of delaying too long. Once the energy and excitement of the crisis has dissipated, it may not matter how many coins are in the piggy bank of credibility. The moment of opportunity for reform may have passed, and if and when the crisis recurs, the agency may be blamed for not having done more.

Boin and colleagues put their finger on the dilemma: "Leaders sit precariously, then, between a rock and a hard place. If they implement crisis prevention, they are chastised for doing too much too soon. If they ignore crisis prevention, they are scolded for having done too little, too late."[10]

The historical examples in this book's first section illustrate the vital role of credibility in setting the stage for policy reform. During both the Elixir Sulfanilamide and thalidomide crises described in Chapters 2 and 3, the U.S. Food and Drug Administration (FDA) mobilized to protect the public. In 1937, the agency sent out every inspector to track down the remaining doses of the dangerous poison. In 1962, after the public came to understand that an agency official had heroically blocked approval of the dangerous drug, the agency's staff scoured the country looking for the thalidomide samples used in research studies that would still pose a risk of severe birth defects. These activities sent the FDA's credibility soaring and allowed the agency's leaders to support legislation to substantially expand its oversight authority.

---

[9] Sharfstein J. JAMA Forum: Flint, Michigan, and the failure of public agencies. 17 February 2016. Accessed June 2, 2017, at https://newsatjama.jama.com/2016/02/17/jama-forum-flint-michigan-and-the-failure-of-public-agencies/.

[10] Boin A, Hart P. Public leadership in times of crisis: Mission impossible? *Public Administration Review*. 2003;63(5):544–553: 546.

In 1976, however, as the Department of Health and Human Services (HHS) was in the midst of bungling its response to the swine flu crisis, it was painfully difficult for the administration to convince Congress to pass basic legislation on liability protection that would allow the vaccine to be available to the public. Indeed, HHS bled so much credibility throughout the course of 1976 that reporters hardly believed any official explanations, and, by October, it took a herculean public relations effort just to respond to erroneous allegations that the vaccine was causing sudden death.

Chapter 5 tells the story of how the FDA's efforts to change its approach to the review of medications to treat HIV infection did not succeed until the arrival of a credible agency leader who had the respect of key advocates, Dr. David Kessler.

The lesson for health agencies is clear: focus on the basics of crisis response, and then, when the iron is hot enough for policy change, strike.

Explaining the Problem

After establishing credibility, health agencies can move to the second part of the public health triple axel: telling a coherent story of what went wrong. This shift to what Boin and colleagues call "meaning making" can be accomplished in stages, as in Maryland's med spa case. The Health Department dropped a single sentence in the initial press release that would become a hook for deeper analysis later.

In identifying the problem, public health leaders should be thoughtful and deliberate. Smith and Elliott distinguish between "first-order" learning, which addresses the proximate causes of problems, and "second order" learning, which asks much deeper questions and "challenges the core organizational paradigm" that may have led to the problem.[11] In other words, leaders should avoid simplistic remedies that fail to provide meaningful solutions by missing the root of the problem.

For an extended period of time in the 1970s and 1980s, British soccer games were vulnerable to crowd stampedes, which frequently led to loss of life. Yet for years, responsible officials treated the problem as "hooliganism," or the tendency of some, often inebriated, fans to act out and create problems around them. The stampedes were generally not recognized as

---

[11] Smith D, Elliott D. Exploring the barriers to learning from crisis: Organizational learning and crisis. *Management Learning*. 2007;38(5):519–538.

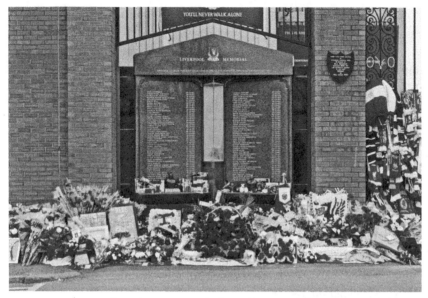

FIGURE 9.1 25 years later, banners outside the stadium recall the Hillsborough tragedy
SOURCE: iStockphoto

the result of failures of planning, stadium structure, crowd control strategy, or game day management. Smith and Elliott noted:

> Despite the lack of a safety culture and serious managerial deficiencies across the country, the persistent belief that the central problem concerned hooliganism (despite significant evidence to the contrary) was key in preventing effective learning. During the pre-crisis stage the emphasis of contingency plans was upon the control of misbehaviour. During crisis events, behavior was frequently misinterpreted as hooliganism, despite contradictory evidence.[12]

These failures culminated in a horrific stampede in April 1989 at Hillsborough Stadium, in which 95 people lost their lives (Figure 9.1).[13] Multiple investigations revealed basic failures in organization and management, demonstrating that the problem was about a lot more than "hooliganism." Soccer organizations and clubs responded by developed systems of tracking, monitoring, and adjusting to changes in crowds.

---

[12] Smith D, Elliott D. Exploring the barriers to learning from crisis: Organizational learning and crisis. *Management Learning.* 2007;38(5):519–538. doi:10.1177/1350507607083205.

[13] The incident remains in the news decades later. Bilefsky D. Six are charged in 1989 Hillsborough stadium disaster in England. *The New York Times.* 28 June 2017.

These systems, which get much closer to the root of the problem, have substantially reduced the risk of hazards to fans.

As in the case of British soccer, it is easy for public officials to fall into the trap of finding a pat answer to the question "What happened?" Major interests, or institutions, may have a vested interest in perpetuating business as usual – making a quick fix and moving on. It takes genuine leadership to look past the comfortable explanations and to delve into major underlying gaps in programs and policy. (Box 9.1).

In such situations, officials can either take a stand themselves or find a lever of change outside the regular course of business.

One such lever is public input. Health agencies can request public comment to create a dialogue around reform, as the Health Department in Maryland chose to do with respect to med spas. In that case, the department feared that the medical community might object to a greater level of regulation and hoped that public comment might create a counterweight to such a parochial interest.[14]

Public comment reflects the absence of a preconceived agenda and demonstrates a willingness to listen. After public comments raise concerns about a sacred cow, the agency can more easily raise questions previously considered taboo. An agency's reasoned response to public comments also allows people to feel heard and demonstrates to all involved the competing pressures facing leadership on a difficult topic.[15]

A second lever of change is the appointment of an independent, expert group to conduct its own assessment. In 2014, for example, Rhode Island Governor Gina Rainmondo asked an expert team at Brown University, supported by a group at Johns Hopkins University, to put together a clear-eyed look at the opioid epidemic. The expert group met with families, addiction treatment providers, and other interested parties and then put forward a report identifying major gaps in the treatment system.[16]

When looking to challenge established thinking about a problem, health officials should recognize that engaging with a small group of experts (and asking them to take public input) is likely to be more

---

[14] In fact, seeing the intense level of public interest, the physician community collaborated on a legislative proposal.

[15] Despite all these advantages, public agencies are often nervous about taking public comment—unnecessarily, in my view.

[16] Rhode Island Governor's Overdose Prevention and Intervention Task Force. Rhode Island's Strategic Plan on Addiction and Overdose. 4 November 2015. Accessed June 2, 2017, at https://www.google.com/url?q=http://www.health.ri.gov/news/temp/RhodeIslandsStrategicPlanOnAddictionAndOverdose.pdf&sa=U&ved=0ahUKEwjjooGTz6DUAhXLQSYKHVKfCpIQFggFMAA&client=internal-uds-cse&usg=AFQjCNEBqaXn30zYn9Mn3dZDCfBEX2P6ig.

BOX 9.1 RESPONDING TO THE NEWTOWN SHOOTINGS

by Governor Martin O'Malley

On December 14, 2012, a 20-year-old brought an assault rifle to Sandy Hook Elementary School. He killed 20 young kindergarten age children and six adults. Was there a more horrific shooting ever in the United States—a wholesale slaughter of innocents?

Immediately, we realized that although tragedy struck Newtown on that day, it could have happened in one of our towns in Maryland on another day. Anyone who has ever sent a child off to school was thinking, "Oh my God, that could have been my kid."

My team had considered developing a legislative strategy on guns after the Aurora shooting in Colorado and then after the shooting at the Sikh temple in Oak Creek, Wisconsin. We had talked about it but not with the same urgency as we did after Newtown. Newtown created a window of opportunity, it created a sense of grief and empathy, and it created a desire to do something.

So I brought together our public safety cabinet, and we compiled a list of all of potential actions in Maryland. My team then picked those items on the list that we thought were both feasible and would actually work.

The next step was to go and round up the votes necessary to pass it. There wasn't a lot of enthusiasm about gun control in the legislature, but we had to put our foot down and insist. I knew it was going to be a huge fight, consume a lot of energy and time, and take a lot of political will. It was really important that we had chosen the evidence-based policies that we thought would work, and this also allowed me to make the argument to the general public.

In addition to finding the votes, we put ourselves into organizing citizens. We held meetings around the state, and we had supportive groups and individuals come down to our State House in Annapolis. The legislators needed to see that there was public support for what we were doing and understand that it wasn't a knee-jerk reaction in the midst of grief.

We avoided vilifying our opponents on the bill. We were constantly praising hunting traditions, and we sent a personalized letter to all of the registered hunters in the state thanking them for hunting and thanking them for paying the registration fee.

Gun legislation was successful in Maryland because there was a truly horrific incident that had occurred. While we acted quickly, we took the time needed to look at the potential impacts and the efficacy of our proposals. We then used every level of political strategy, from working with individual legislators, mobilizing supporters, and communicating directly with potential opposition, to move the bill forward.

effective than calling together a large, unwieldy group of "stakeholders" whose members may be focused on their own interests. (See Appendix 3: Banishing Stakeholders).

Indeed, Rhode Island's thorough, independent review of the opioid crisis led to creative new efforts to expand evidence-based treatment in centers of excellence and in the detention system. The *Providence Journal* called Governor Raimondo's plan "a smart, multi-pronged plan to attack the drug-overdose deaths afflicting Rhode Island" that "should help to slow what has become a devastating loss of lives."[17]

A third lever may be found internal to an agency—in career officials with impeccable reputations. In 2009, for example, the FDA faced a crisis caused by the use of highly irregular procedures in its clearance of a device to treat injured knees. *The Wall Street Journal* had published a series of reports about the unusual involvement of the Office of the Commissioner in what typically would be handled by the Center for Devices and Radiological Health.[18] The reports suggested that the commissioner might have become involved in pushing for a device's approval following political pressure.

Facing a crisis that called into question the integrity of its decision-making, the agency asked three senior agency officials to assess what happened. The ensuing report, which found fundamental failures in the device review process, was widely reported.[19] *The New York Times* noted, "The agency has never before publicly questioned the process behind one of its approvals, never admitted that a regulatory decision was influenced by politics, and never accused a former commissioner of questionable conduct."[20] The report became the basis for a series of reforms led by the Center for Devices and Radiological Health.

Regardless of whether an agency seeks outside input or tackles the cause of a crisis itself, it is vital that assessments be well written, clearly presented, and understandable. This generally means including an executive summary, the credentials and methods of those engaged, and a clear explanation of key findings.

---

[17] Editorial: Rhode Island faces the opioid crisis. *Providence Journal.* 18 May 2016. In late 2017, Rhode Island reported a decline in opioid overdose deaths.
[18] Chittum R. WSJ exposes corruption at the FDA. *Columbia Journalism Review.* 6 March 2009. Accessed June 2, 2017, at http://archives.cjr.org/the_audit/wsj_exposes_corruption_at_the.php.
[19] Harris G, Halbfinger DM. FDA reveals it fell to a push by lawmakers. *The New York Times.* 24 September 2009.
[20] Harris G, Halbfinger DM. FDA reveals it fell to a push by lawmakers. *The New York Times.* 24 September 2009.

When issued during or shortly after a crisis by a public health agency with credibility, a well-done report can shape public thinking about the underlying problem—and bring attention to much-needed reform.[21]

Proposing and Fighting for Specific and Realistic Solutions

Developing an effective strategy for policy change—the third part of the triple axel—involves considering alternative viewpoints, balancing the ideal with the realistic, and then fighting for progress.

Before settling on an action plan, officials should always consider ideas contrary to the prevailing wisdom. One reason is, of course, that ideas outside the usual frame of reference might have some value. A second reason is to assure those who will disagree with the plan that their perspective was taken into account. As Boin and Hart have written, "Leaders should not push reform without considering opposite arguments. If they use the crisis to ignore critics, they will mobilize their own opposition at a time when their performance is already under scrutiny."[22]

Plans must also be realistic. It is not helpful to propose a set of activities that has no chance of adoption and thus to forego opportunities to make meaningful progress that generate momentum for further reform. Where to draw the line, of course, is a critical matter of judgment for health leaders (Box 9.2).

Realistic plans typically require compromise—the acceptance of the fact that there may be a path not taken, a goal that could not be reached. Figuring out what constitutes a smart compromise is the essence of political strategy.[23] Health leaders should consult with people savvy about local politics to figure out what goals are sensible as part of a reorientation during a crisis to longer-term solutions. (See Appendix 7: On Working for Henry Waxman.)

Once a strategy is set, public health leaders can roll up their sleeves to make the case for change. Success may well require calling key decision-makers, working with reporters, writing op/eds, and developing alliances with key advocates in the public and private sectors. A key goal is to

---

[21] A classic example is the U.S. Department of Agriculture's report to Congress after the Sulfanilamide crisis, described in Chapter 2.

[22] Boin A, Hart P. Public Leadership in times of crisis: Mission impossible? *Public Administration Review.* 2003;63(5):544–553: 551.

[23] Sharfstein J. On working for Henry Waxman. *Milbank Quarterly.* 2014;92:186–190.

BOX 9.2 OPPORTUNITY IN CRISIS: JACK IN THE BOX AND USDA

by Grace Mandel

In December 1992, four children died from eating hamburgers at Jack in the Box, a fast-food restaurant. By the end of the crisis, over 700 people had fallen ill due to the contaminated hamburgers.

At first, blame focused squarely on the Jack in Box corporation, which sold hamburgers contaminated with E. Coli O157:H7. Soon, however, questions began to be directed to the federal agency responsible for meat safety, the U.S. Department of Agriculture (USDA). While acknowledging that it failed to cook its hamburgers to standards set in the state of Washington, Jack in the Box claimed to have used the temperature specified by USDA standards, a temperature too low to kill the E. Coli bacteria.

The newly appointed Secretary of Agriculture, Mike Epsy, seized on the outbreak as an opportunity to improve food safety. The USDA soon changed the temperature recommendations for raw meat and required "safe handling" labels of raw meat and poultry. The changes in cooking temperatures was a politically easy solution to the crisis. The fast-food industry was looking for new standards to help reassure consumer that their products were safe. The beef industry, which had long opposed more regulation, also reversed their position on food temperature. A beef industry representative was quoted, "The coverage, so far, has focused on cooking procedures at the fast food outlet, not the beef industry issues. Let's try to keep it that way."[1] Epsy could have decided to stop there.

But he went further. In addition to the food cooking and labeling requirements, the USDA decided to classify E. Coli O157:H7 as an adulterant, meaning that beef contaminated with E. Coli O157:H7 could no longer be legally sold. Espy said, "USDA will be making a decisive break from the past. In the future, USDA will not wait for pathogens to become a problem . . . USDA will strive to reduce contamination from the farm to table."[2]

The beef industry sued the USDA to stop the change. This time, however, an advocacy group formed by parents of E. Coli victims fought back. The grieving father of three-year old Riley Detwiler, one of the children who died after eating a Jack in the Box hamburger, appeared on *Oprah* and CNN and advocated for food safety.[3] He also participated in a televised town hall meeting, where he asked President Clinton personally to improve meat inspection standards. The USDA implemented the new standards, and, since that time, the percentage of ground beef contaminated with E. Coli has declined by 80%.[4]

---

[1] Nestle, M. *Safe Food: The Politics of Food Safety*. Berkeley: University of California Press, 2010: 84.
[2] Fox N. *Spoiled: The Dangerous Truth about a Food Chain Gone Haywire*. New York: Basic Books, 1997.
[3] King W. E. Coli victim leaves legacy of awareness. *The Seattle Times*. 25 February 1993.
[4] Andrews J. Jack in the Box and the decline of E. Coli. *Food Safety News*. 11 February 2013.

counter competing narratives and explain why other solutions will not work. Boin and Hart set out the challenge:

> Reform leaders in particular have much persuading to do because their plans differ markedly from what exists. They have to convince multiple audiences that what they want is good, realistic, and inevitable. Moreover, they must convince stakeholders that the benefits of the proposed reform outweigh the sunk costs of existing structures and policies. This requires not only effective command and selection of facts but also the rhetorical skills to present them. It also touches on the socioemotional bond between leaders and citizens. Leaders need to do more than expose a crisis; they also need to reassure followers they know the right (if not the only) way out. Reformist crisis leaders, therefore, need to be constructive and destructive at the same time: build up their case for change, burn down the bridges to the past, and disqualify competing policy alternatives.[24]

This is all a lot to ask of a health leader at a time of stress for his or her agency and community, which is perhaps why few health leaders try to capitalize on opportunities created by crisis. Many see such battles as too difficult or too political, and, in some cases, they may be right. Yet health leaders who shy away from reform during pivotal moments may be fore-going major advances for public health.

Such a moment came several years ago in California, in the midst of a major measles outbreak that involved Disneyland. Some suggested that because of growing opposition to vaccine mandates, there was no chance the crisis could lead to longstanding reform. Others thought there was a real opening for change. (See Appendix 6: Of Mouse and Measles.) In the end, public health officials and elected leaders led by state senator and pediatrician Richard Pan led a successful coalition in support of adopt stronger vaccine requirements for schools.[25]

Rather than assume change is too hard to achieve, leaders can work on developing the skills to develop and fight for needed reforms. Then, at a time of maximum agency credibility, leaders can make a straightforward case: here's the crisis, here's what caused it, and here's what we need to do to reduce the chance of another crisis in the future.

---

[24] Boin A, Hart P. Public leadership in times of crisis: Mission impossible? *Public Administration Review*. 2003;63(5):544–553: 550.

[25] Martinez M, Watts A. California governor signs vaccine bill that bans personal, religious exemptions. CNN. 30 June 2015.

In the case of Maryland's outbreak of "flesh eating" bacteria, the Health Department pointed to severe injuries and deaths in a cosmetic surgery clinic, to harm caused by sloppy medical care in the absence of oversight, and to the need for a licensure system to protect the public. It certainly helped that outside, credible patient safety experts echoed this assessment, and that advocates pushed for legislative change alongside health leaders. No one said the triple axel was easy, but landing one under pressure is golden.

III |Strategic Considerations

T HIS FINAL SECTION TACKLES two topics about crisis strategy that are rarely covered in formal public health training. Chapter 11 is about responsibility and blame. Culpability figures prominently in the aftermath of crisis, and a strategic approach can help health officials weather the storm. Chapter 12 provides a perspective on how leaders can purposefully awaken a sense of crisis to address significant health threats in their communities. Jumping with two feet into crisis certainly carries risks. But it also can lead to remarkable achievements for public health.

10 | Responsibility and Blame

AS SECRETARY OF MARYLAND'S DEPARTMENT of Health and Mental Hygiene, I developed a routine to unwind at the end of the week. After packing my bag for home, I would sit back down at my desk and click through the major headlines of a few newspapers. One hot summer evening, my eye was naturally drawn to a front-page story in *The Washington Post* about a new policy issued by some health department somewhere that strongly discouraged camp counselors from helping campers with sunscreen. According to the article, the policy also strictly forbade one camper from applying sunscreen to another.

"The rules are 'absurd,'" one dermatologist was quoted as saying. "This is the biggest known carcinogen that children are exposed to. We should be asking camp counselors to take an active role in promoting skin protection."[1]

Chuckling to myself, I wondered which unfortunate agency had issued this policy. I stopped chuckling a few paragraphs later when I realized that the agency was my own.

I tracked down the division director who had sent out the new orders.

"Josh, give me one example where it might be appropriate for one camper to help another with sunscreen?" he asked.

"Siblings!" I responded. "Best friends forever!"

"Okay," he replied.

Now we faced a choice. Should we plod on forward without admitting error, having issued the policy, or should we retract it? And could this wait until Monday morning? I imagined explaining the situation to the governor and took a deep breath.

---

[1] Fisher M. Md. to require parental permission before kids can use sunscreen. *The Washington Post.* 1 July 2011.

I tracked down our department's communications director, who had left the office hours ago. She cheerfully informed me she was leaving in the morning to go camping "off the grid." I responded that, unfortunately, she was needed for media inquiries the entire weekend—unless she could explain to *The Washington Post* editors in the next hour that we had made a mistake and were retracting the policy. A normally mild-mannered, calm person, she sprang into action. Within minutes, the online story read, "Maryland health officials were making revisions late Friday night to a new policy that would have severely restricted who could apply sunscreen to children attending summer camps."

The next day, the *Post*'s story was titled, "Maryland Officials Scrap New Sunscreen Restrictions." The article began:

> Less than a day after dermatologists and parents said Maryland's new policy on sunscreen at summer camps would make it far more likely that children would suffer skin damage, the state health department Saturday scrapped all of the restrictions it had imposed just three weeks ago.
>
> The new policy, announced in a statement that noted in bold capital letters that it "supersedes all previous interpretive memoranda regarding sunscreen," will no longer direct camps to steer counselors away from helping children apply sunscreen. It also removes any mention of the previous ban on children assisting each other in putting on sunscreen.[2]

Our communications director went camping.

The episode was humiliating, and the natural inclination was to hope no one read the paper that weekend. Over the next few months, however, I found myself telling the sunscreen story again and again to different audiences, as demonstration of the fact that I recognized my agency could make errors and that we would be responsive to real concerns. "If you don't believe me that we can change our mind," I would say, "Just ask campers whether they are allowed to use sunscreen."

Issues of responsibility and blame, apologies or apologia, are rarely discussed in public health trainings. But they are seldom forgotten in practice.[3] That is because, in the blunt words of Boin and Hart, "Post-crisis

---

[2] Fisher M. Maryland officials scrap new sunscreen restrictions. *The Washington Post.* 2 July 2011.
[3] Nor is it forgotten at gatherings of public health officials. That's where I shared stories of sunscreen regulations run amok, and I learned how New York labeled whiffle ball and freeze tag contact sports. See Neporent L. New York Health Department will no longer regulate fun. ABCNews.com. 19 April 2011.

investigations are less about learning than they are about blaming."[4] There will be blame, and leaders of health agencies should be able to think strategically about how to handle such accusations before faced with the pain of dealing with them. Boin and Hart continued:

> Postmortem investigations often unveil erroneous policies or bureaucratic mismanagement. This erosion of public trust in the capability of state institutions to perform their classic custodial functions is accompanied by increasingly assertive and tenacious media coverage of risks, disasters, and other critical events. The aftermath of today's crises tends to be as intense and contentious as the acute crisis periods are, with leaders put under pressure by streams of informal investigations, proactive journalism, insurance claims and juridical (including criminal) proceedings against them. Leadership in the face of this sort of adversity is, in short, precarious.[5]

In this hostile environment, the natural tendency is to duck and cover—to try to avoid blame at all costs. This might be called the "it wasn't me" strategy, based on the hit single in 2000 by the recording artist Shaggy.[6]

Resolute denial has one clear advantage: It allows officials to stay on message about the agency's response, at least temporarily. Unfortunately, if and when the public realizes that the agency was, at least in part, responsible for what happened, the result can be a drain of credibility—and the end of the line for agency leaders. Indeed, by the end, the "it wasn't me" strategy did not even make sense to the protagonist in Shaggy's song.[7]

A better approach is for health officials to consider the true role that the agency might have played in causing or contributing to a crisis and then, based on this assessment, to make strategic decisions about accepting responsibility in a difficult and often adversarial environment.

---

[4] Boin A, Hart P. Public leadership in times of crisis: Mission impossible? *Public Administration Review.* 2003;63(5):544–553: 548.

[5] Boin A, Hart P. Public leadership in times of crisis: Mission impossible? *Public Administration Review.* 2003;63(5):544–553: 545.

[6] In the song, after a young man who was caught *in flagrante delicto* by his girlfriend despairs on how to handle the situation, his friend advises, "To be a true player you have to know how to play . . . never admit to a word when she say/Makes a claim and you tell her, baby no way."

[7] He sings: "We should tell her that I'm sorry/for the pain that I've caused/You may think that you're a player/But you're completely lost."

Not the Agency's Fault

When a health official is sure that his or her agency bears no responsibility for a crisis, a world of potential for communications opens up. During the crisis response, the agency can stretch its wings and make the case for the vital role of public health.

I stumbled onto this opportunity in my first days as Health Commissioner in Baltimore in mid-December 2005. Just two weeks away, on January 1, 2006, Medicare was going to implement a new prescription drug benefit, known as Medicare Part D. The new program was a step forward for health; after more than 35 years, the Medicare program would finally cover much of the cost of prescription drugs for tens of millions of our nation's older adults.

However, as part of the legislative deal that made Part D possible, Congress had made the decision to upend the prescription drug coverage for a particularly vulnerable population: older adults poor enough to qualify for Medicaid as well as Medicare. Prior to January 1, 2016, these individuals enjoyed comprehensive drug coverage through Medicaid, which allowed them to go to any pharmacy for all their medications. At midnight on January 1, 2016, however, their coverage would transition to private insurance plans in the Medicare Part D program—plans that might not cover their usual medications or allow them to pick up their prescriptions at their usual pharmacies.

In Baltimore, about 28,000 vulnerable citizens had coverage through both Medicare and Medicaid. Each one would need to navigate the January 1 transition successfully or risk losing access to essential medications for diabetes, mental illness, seizure disorders, or other serious conditions. I feared that even a small amount of trouble figuring out the new system could lead to great harm.[8]

This was not a crisis of the Health Department's making. But I challenged my new staff to think about solutions. At first, we considered setting up a hotline for older adults affected by the transition. But this idea raised several practical difficulties, including how many people we would need to staff the hotline, and what we could really do to help people.

Then one of the senior staff pointed out that there are only about 125 pharmacies in Baltimore. After the clock struck midnight on January 1, older adults running into problems would literally be standing in pharmacies, unable to get their medicines. She asked: what if we worked

---

[8] Salganik MW. City to aid Medicare launch; Health agency to monitor seniors' needs as drug plans shift. *The Baltimore Sun.* 21 December 2005.

with the city's pharmacies to provide technical support and, if needed, emergency funding for prescriptions during a transitional period? I quickly secured a commitment of about $100,000 from my new boss, Mayor Martin O'Malley, to pay for the project.

That's how, by my third week on the job, the Health Department came to set up a 24-hour surveillance system through local pharmacies to identify people who were unable to receive their essential medications under their new coverage. Just before the start of the new year, I held a press conference with the mayor to warn people about the potential disruption of Medicare Part D implementation. *The Baltimore Sun* reported:

> Baltimore City Health Department will announce today that it will set up a 24-hour system to ensure that thousands of low-income elderly and disabled will get needed medicines as they are switched from state-run programs to the new Medicare drug plan Jan. 1. The new system will monitor problems and help resolve them quickly, Dr. Joshua Sharfstein, the city's health commissioner, said yesterday. In urgent cases, the city will pay for prescriptions to be filled to ensure an uninterrupted supply, but more often he expects the city will help people to enroll for the benefit or pharmacists to resolve billing problems.[9]

One of my key messages was the need for public health engagement in an issue outside our usual domain. The initial story quoted me as saying, "If one person switches, it's an insurance issue. When 28,000 people switch on one day, it's a public health issue."

On January 1, the Centers for Medicare and Medicaid Services flipped the switch on the new system, and we waited. Within minutes, calls started coming from pharmacies to our hotline. We helped pharmacists navigate through the new system and promised backup funds when needed. We tracked emergency department visits as outcome measures. Our efforts helped send the message that the Health Department was in the business of protecting the most vulnerable people in our city.[10] The mayor was thrilled by positive attention from the national media, and the staff were energized.[11]

---

[9] Salganik MW. City to aid Medicare launch; Health agency to monitor seniors' needs as drug plans shift. *The Baltimore Sun*. 21 December 2005.

[10] O'Keefe G, Veal L, Marisa N, Goetzinger K, Stewart J, Sharfstein JM. A public health response to implementation of Medicare Part D. *Public Health Reports*. 2007 Jan-Feb;122(1):101–104.

[11] We did run into one problem: Frustration from other elected officials that we had not involved them in the initial announcement. My apologies and explanations that I had no idea whether this would be successful were not particularly effective. But I involved them in future responses to good effect.

During this period, reporters often asked who I blamed for the problem: Congress for passing the law or the Centers for Medicare and Medicaid Services for messing up the implementation? I demurred, noting where possible that prescription drug coverage was a positive step for the health of older adults. My goal was to keep communication lines open with the Medicare program to provide the best service to older adults in Baltimore. I avoided pointing a finger to keep the focus on what we were doing to help people in the city during a rocky transition.

In retrospect, it's hard for me to imagine a better start to my work at a public health agency. Even now, a dozen years later, people in Baltimore still stop me on the street to tell me how much they appreciated the city's efforts at that time. Many still say that they never expected the Health Department to have been involved in helping Medicare patients in the first place.

A decade later, a new health commissioner in Baltimore also began to make her reputation in the city by rising to a challenge not of her agency's making. Dr. Leana Wen is a physician in her early 30s with a specialty in emergency medicine and a boundless enthusiasm for public health. When protests and civil unrest destroyed several pharmacies in Baltimore in the spring of 2015, she was just weeks into the job. Nonetheless, she moved swiftly to respond. As Kevin Rector of *The Baltimore Sun* reported:

> The department created a hotline for people to call for assistance filling prescriptions. It blasted out information on social media. And when it realized older people most in need weren't getting those messages, its staff "walked door to door." The department sent "informational letters to all physicians in the state" informing them how they could help, and eventually distributed more than 200 prescriptions directly to the most vulnerable residents.[12]

Dr. Wen herself was featured in several news reports talking about her first-hand work on the challenges facing the city. In an article published later with the city's chief medical officer, she explained why the Health Department jumped into action: "This was what we called a 'code' in the hospital: an emergency scenario with an acute situation requiring an immediate and coordinated response."[13]

---

[12] Rector K. TCA Regional News. 23 December 2015.

[13] Wen LS, Warren KE, Tay S, Khaldun JS, O'Neill DL, Farrow OD. Public health in the unrest: Baltimore's preparedness and response after Freddie Gray's death. *American Journal of Public Health.* 2015 Oct;105(10):1957–1959.

After the unrest had subsided, Dr. Wen used her elevated profile to call attention to core inequities in access to jobs, housing, and education.[14] She focused her planning efforts on expanding services for individuals suffering from trauma and in developing public health solutions for violence.[15] The Health Department was able to garner more than $10 million in grants to develop programs to promote this vision. And Dr. Wen has yet to slow down since.[16]

These experiences exemplify opportunity in crisis—not just to solve a problem but to build the reputation of a public health agency and to construct a foundation for further progress in the future.

Your Fault

Unfortunately, for every story of a health agency coming to the rescue, there is a crisis that is largely or entirely its own fault. Once any leader realizes the problem is self-inflicted, the first instinct may be to stay very quiet and hope nobody notices. The second instinct may be to blame others. The business literature includes a taxonomy of 11 ways to not say you are sorry (Table 10.1).

Trying to evade responsibility, however, can be a fool's errand. Just look at what happened to the many public officials involved in the Flint, Michigan, water crisis. In 2014, after city officials made the fateful decision to switch the source of the municipal water supply, environmental officials failed to require corrosion control measures. The Flint water was discolored, malodorous, contaminated with *Legionella* bacteria, and poisoned with lead. Had the problem been recognized and remediated quickly, little harm would have resulted. Yet the inability of multiple agencies to recognize this mistake, take responsibility, and fix it led to more than a year of delays, exposure of thousands of children to high levels of lead, and several deaths from *Legionella*.

In the face of complaints about the look, taste, and smell of the water, local and state officials responded by denying there were problems with safety—even as some brought bottled water into their own headquarters. Then, when

---

[14] Wen LS, Sharfstein JM. Unrest in Baltimore: The role of public health. *Journal of the American Medical Association.* 2015 Jun 23–30;313(24):2425–2426.

[15] Wen LS, Warren KE, Tay S, Khaldun JS, O'Neill DL, Farrow OD. Public health in the unrest: Baltimore's preparedness and response after Freddie Gray's death. *American Journal of Public Health.* 2015 Oct;105(10):1957–1959.

[16] Khazan O. Working a million hours a day to heal a city. *The Atlantic.* 22 June 2015.

TABLE 10.1 Selected Corporate Image Restoration Strategies

STRATEGY	KEY CHARACTERISTIC
Simple Denial	Did not perform act
Shift the Blame	Act performed by another
Provocation	Responded to act of another
Defeasibility	Lack of information or ability
Accident	Act was a mishap
Good Intentions	Meant well in act
Bolstering	Stress good traits
Minimization	Act not serious
Differentiation	Act less offensive
Transcendence	More important considerations
Attack Accuser	Reduce credibility of accuser

Source: Benoit L. Image repair discourse and crisis communication. *Public Relations Review* 1997;23(2);177–186.

a scientist at the Environmental Protection Agency (EPA) wrote a draft report sounding the alarm about lead poisoning, the head of the agency's regional office undermined the draft and passed the buck to the state's environmental agency. On July 1, 2015, the EPA regional director wrote to the Flint mayor:

> The preliminary draft report should not have been released outside the agency. . . . When the report has been revised and fully vetted by EPA management, the findings and recommendations will be shared with the city and [the Michigan Department of Environmental Quality] will be responsible for following up with the city.[17]

Later in 2015, an outside expert in water quality, Professor Marc Edwards of Virginia Tech University, came to Flint. He noted the lack of a corrosion control plan and tested the water. When, in September, he found high levels of lead, a spokesman for the state environmental agency responded with additional denials. He told a journalist:

> It's scientifically probable a research team that specializes in looking for lead in water could have found it in Flint when the city was on its old water supply. We won't know that, because they've only just arrived in town

---

[17] Lynch J. EPA stayed silent on Flint's tainted water. *Detroit News.* 12 January 2016.

and quickly proven the theory they set out to prove, and while the state appreciates academic participation in this discussion, offering broad, dire public health advice based on some quick testing could be seen as fanning political flames irresponsibly. Residents of Flint concerned about the health of their community don't need more of that.[18]

Finally, a local pediatrician, Dr. Mona Hanna-Attisha, conducted her own analysis and found substantial increases in lead poisoning in areas of the city with high lead levels. Yet, even then, the state health director wrote his staff, "I would like to make a strong statement with a demonstration of proof that the lead blood levels seen are not out of the ordinary and are attributable to seasonal fluctuations."[19] At a press conference with the governor, the health director publicly minimized the problem, leading the heroic Dr. Hanna-Attisha to shake her head "no" in front of the cameras. "I've always had trouble keeping a poker face," she told television host Rachel Maddow.[20]

Why did it take so incredibly long for any official to accept there was a problem, take responsibility, and do whatever was possible to fix the problem? A subsequent independent review of the Flint debacle found "government failure, intransigence, unpreparedness, delay, inaction, and environmental injustice."[21] Even in the face of overwhelming evidence, officials failed to accept what was happening, perhaps because doing so would mean accepting responsibility (Figure 10.1).

If so, this was a disastrous strategy, both for the public officials and for public health. The consequences, external scrutiny, and public anger grew exponentially. The result was one of the largest crises facing health agencies in memory. After the dust settled, the Michigan attorney general charged multiple health and environmental officials, including the state health director, with crimes for their roles in Flint.[22] (See Appendix 4: Flint, Michigan, and the Failure of Public Agencies.)

---

[18] Kennedy M. Lead-laced water In Flint: A step-by-step look at the makings of a crisis. National Public Radio. 20 April 2016.

[19] Fonger R. Manslaughter charge reaches Gov. Snyder's cabinet over Flint water crisis. *Mlive.* 14 June 2017. Accessed June 20, 2017, at http://www.mlive.com/news/flint/index.ssf/2017/06/two. html.

[20] Fonger R. Crusading doctor shakes head "no" at Gov. Snyder's Flint news conference. *Mlive.* 14 January 2016. Accessed June 20, 2017, at http://www.mlive.com/news/flint/index.ssf/2016/01/ hurley_doctor_says_she_couldnt.html.

[21] Flint Water Advisory Task Force: Final Report. March 2016. Accessed June 11, 2017, at https:// www.michigan.gov/documents/snyder/FWATF_FINAL_REPORT_21March2016_517805_7.pdf.

[22] Atkinson S, Davey M. 5 charged with involuntary manslaughter in Flint water crisis. *The New York Times.* 14 June 2017.

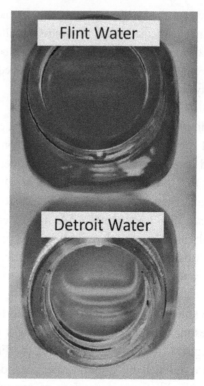

FIGURE 10.1 Flint water compared to Detroit water
Courtesy flintwaterstudy.org

The polar opposite of the Flint model is for health leaders to move as quickly as possible to fix problems, taking responsibility as needed along the way. As Ralph Tyler, the chief lawyer for Baltimore, used to tell me in his deep, and compelling voice, "When answering for a mistake, nothing is better than starting with 'It's fixed.'"

"It's fixed" beats blaming others, promising to investigate, setting deadlines for a response, and every other possible thing to say. And when it is fixed, a health official can, in the second sentence, accept responsibility if appropriate and come out stronger for having done so.

This is true even if the facts of the situation are quite embarrassing, as in the case of Maryland's sunscreen policy. Of course, the challenge of accepting responsibility becomes much more serious, as in Flint, when agency errors cause or threaten to cause real harm and when immediate fixes are not possible.

Soon after I started as secretary in Maryland, I had my own brush with an error related to childhood lead poisoning, three years before Flint. Soon after I had taken office, I learned that the directors of our state's laboratory had destroyed thousands of children's lead test results.

How bad was it? The laboratory's leadership had apparently ordered a shredding machine to be backed up to the Health Department's building and hoisted boxes of records into the shredder for destruction. They then apparently attempted to wipe clean the computer to eliminate the backup copies of the records. Why? They were apparently frustrated with having answering requests for records from lawyers suing landlords on behalf of children. Of course, the actions created a risk that these plaintiffs' attorneys—and the children who were their clients—would not be able to access the evidence of harm that was needed for their clients' cases.

I suppose I could have responded by denying anything was wrong, or pointing out that it was likely that another agency had copies of the records. Instead, as soon as I heard what had happened, I quickly recognized this situation as a crisis for our department—one that was entirely our own fault. I called one of the plaintiff's attorneys involved, who I happened to know from jury service years earlier, and owned up to what had happened. He was stunned and angry. I then asked him to convene all the involved attorneys the next day.

I started that memorable meeting by accepting responsibility on behalf of the department and personally apologizing. I told the lawyers of my initial actions, and I promised to keep them informed as we took additional steps to fix the problem. As soon as the meeting ended, I went back to my office and called a local reporter myself. The next day, *The Baltimore Sun's* news story read:

> The state's health secretary said Friday that his department's laboratory has destroyed test results dating back to the 1980s documenting lead poisoning of Maryland children—potentially thousands of records that plaintiffs' lawyers say are crucial to pursuing lawsuits seeking damages on behalf of poisoned children and their families.
>
> Dr. Joshua Sharfstein said he has asked for an investigation of how the destruction of records happened, replaced the lab's director and ordered efforts be made to recover whatever test results might have been deleted from state computer files.
>
> "We regret this, and we're going to do everything possible to make it right," Sharfstein said in a telephone interview.[23]

---

[23] Wheeler T. Health department investigating destruction of lead paint records. *The Baltimore Sun.* 12 March 2011.

The crisis lingered for a few more weeks, until we had recovered electronic copies of the records (an enormous relief) and taken other corrective action.[24] Our department's inspector general played a helpful role by providing an independent assessment of what had gone wrong. By unequivocally and proactively accepting responsibility early, and by taking quick action to address the problem, I was able to maintain the credibility to see the situation through.

It is never easy to say you are sorry. It's particularly difficult in an adversarial political climate. But the alternative to apology when an agency is wholly responsible for a problem seldom involves skating through the crisis untouched. The alternative is most likely derision, disrespect, and a loss of credibility, even among friends and allies. Admitting an error quickly and decisively is not a guaranteed strategy. But it can upend expectations, preserve trust, and help public health officials to survive to fight another day.

Partly Your Fault

The greatest test of communications and strategy comes after a health official realizes that a crisis is partly, but not entirely, the responsibility of his or her agency. On the one hand, disavowing all responsibility and claiming to be coming to the rescue is risky, because of the likelihood the agency will be tagged with some of the blame. On the other hand, accepting all responsibility may be unfair and frustrating to agency staff and can complicate the response. In this difficult scenario, public health officials often feel trapped between participating in a cover-up and admitting incompetence without justification. Threading the needle between these extremes requires consideration of several different strategies, each of which has advantages and disadvantages.

Shift Responsibility

One approach is to try to push the lion's share of culpability to others. If successful, this strategy can avoid unnecessary harm to the agency's reputation and position health officials to propose solutions to address the problem. However, pointing the finger at others is a risky maneuver that can backfire.

---

[24] Calvert S. Officials: Md. health lab improving after lead records tumult. *The Baltimore Sun.* 4 June 2011.

Success in the blame game is most likely when the agency truly bears minimal responsibility, when the response is swift, and when there are credible external voices supporting the health official's story. But playing this game is not for the faint of heart.

In May 2010, while working at the U.S. Food and Drug Administration (FDA), I watched and listened as a representative from the dietary supplement industry testified before the Special Committee on Aging of the U.S. Senate. The topic of the hearing was a report from the Government Accountability Office finding that many dietary supplements were marketed with claims, such as "cures cancer," that are illegal under the Food, Drug and Cosmetic Act. One purpose of the hearing for the Senators was to figure out who to blame.

I was sitting in the front row of the hearing room, because I was to be a witness on the second panel.

Midway through first panel, Tennessee Senator Bob Corker asked the industry witness whether either the FDA or the Federal Trade Commission should have identified the illegal claims before the products went on the market. "So," he asked the industry representative, "[The FDA is] not carrying out their responsibilities in that regard. Is that correct?" The witness responded, "Yes, sir."[25]

I was stunned by this answer. Under federal law, the FDA simply does not have the authority to review claims before marketing, so it was not fair to expect the agency to have caught the problem ahead of time. In theory, it might have been possible for the FDA to have found some of the suspect products soon after coming onto the market. But in practice, with minimal resources, there was no way the agency could have done so. So as this line of questioning was developing, subconsciously, I began shaking my head.

And Senator Corker noticed.

What came next happened so quickly and unexpectedly that I am not able to tell the story from memory. Fortunately, the U.S. Senate keeps official transcripts of its hearings. The transcript of this hearing captures the senator looking up from the panel of witnesses, and saying: "Somebody behind you is shaking their head, 'No, no, no'—I don't know which one of you is right."[26]

---

[25] Hearing before the Special Committee on Aging, U.S. Senate. *Dietary supplements: What seniors need to know*. 26 May 2010. Serial 111–118. Washington, DC: Government Printing Office, 2010: 92.

[26] Hearing before the Special Committee on Aging, U.S. Senate. *Dietary supplements: What seniors need to know*. 26 May 2010. Serial 111–118. Washington, DC: Government Printing Office, 2010: 92.

Soon after, Senator Corker received a note from his staff and added:

> I understand the gentleman who was shaking his head vigorously in the background is our next witness, the FDA or part of the FDA, saying that in fact, it is not their responsibility, if his body language is correct, to actually check the labels. Before you leave the dais, do you want to say anything else about that? Apparently he feels 180 degrees the opposite. I find that kind of odd.[27]

In terms of the etiquette of Congressional hearings, this was like my arriving to testify without wearing pants. But as a matter of law, I was on solid ground. The industry witness quickly conceded "there is no preapproval process," and, when I testified,[28] Senator Corker said he recognized the difficult situation that the agency faced.

While I somehow managed to seek my way through this time, the strategy of forcefully pushing responsibility elsewhere holds two major risks. The first is that in the midst of a crisis, the aggrieved party may resent the action and become less willing to assist in the response. This is a particularly important consideration when multiple government agencies share the blame. Pointing to a sister agency as being responsible is an especially dangerous move if that agency's collaboration is essential to the solution.

The second risk is that the strategy comes across as an insincere attempt to dodge deserved responsibility. In September 2014, the deputy administrator of the National Highway Transportation Safety Agency testified in Congress in the wake of revelations that a defective ignition switch in the Chevrolet Cobalt had led to at least 19 deaths. His plan was simple: Blame the manufacturer, General Motors. He testified that his agency "was actively trying to find the ball," while General Motors, "was actively trying to hide the ball."[29]

---

[27] Hearing before the Special Committee on Aging, U.S. Senate. *Dietary supplements: What seniors need to know*. 26 May 2010. Serial 111–118. Washington, DC: Government Printing Office, 2010: 95.

[28] To diffuse the awkwardness of the situation, I added to my oral testimony, "I apologize for shaking my head. [FDA Commissioner] Dr. Hamburg has told me I should not give up my day job to become a poker player." Hearing before the Special Committee on Aging, U.S. Senate. *Dietary supplements: What seniors need to know*. 26 May 2010. Serial 111–118. Washington, DC: Government Printing Office, 2010: 99.

[29] Stout H, Kessler AM. Senators take auto agency to task over G.M. recall. *The New York Times*. 16 September 2014.

This message was not well received. Instead of focusing on the company, both Democratic and Republican senators lashed out at the agency, arguing that it "failed to use its full authority over automakers and that it did not figure out defect trends that consumers themselves had alerted the agency to." Senator Claire McCaskill, a Democrat from Missouri, said to the deputy administrator:

> You want to obfuscate responsibility, rather than take responsibility. We've all said shame on [General Motors]. You've got to take some responsibility that this isn't being handled correctly.

When dodging responsibility inflames key audiences, the result can be anger out of proportion to the agency's share of the blame.

Fake It Until You Make It

An alternative to engaging in a discussion about blame or responsibility is for agencies to limit messaging to being " focused on fixing the problem." The goal of this approach is to delay the day of reckoning until the problem is fixed.

This strategy is naturally appealing in a highly politicized environment, where accepting blame early can lead to a frenzy of allegations that can complicate the crisis response. The likelihood of success in holding off tough questions, however, dwindles as it takes longer and longer to fix the problem. If a problem can be remedied in a few hours or days, then it is reasonable for an agency to keep its eyes facing forward. But as weeks drag into months, and a crisis lingers, this strategy begins to look to the world like an attempt to evade blame.

I learned this difficult lesson during the implementation of the Affordable Care Act, when I served as chair of the board of Maryland's health insurance exchange. After October 1, 2013, when our exchange (like several others) crashed out of the gate, there was little appetite to discuss responsibility for problems; we poured all our efforts into trying to fix it. Four months in, however, we still had not told any story of what had happened, leaving us vulnerable to the allegations it was all our fault. It was not a high point for me when one commentator in *The Washington Post* wrote, "Hubris, vanity and plain incompetence . . . have cost tens of thousands of Marylanders health coverage for months."[30]

---

[30] Dvorak P. Maryland's health insurance-site debacle: A scandal of incompetence. *The Washington Post.* 13 January 2014.

This scathing criticism had two parts: first, we were arrogant, vain, and incompetent. Second, "tens of thousands of Marylanders" had lost coverage as a result. Fortunately, this latter accusation was untrue; we set up a backup system that would (and did) assure access to insurance. The "hubris, vanity and plain incompetence" part, however, was difficult to counter, even though we knew that what had gone wrong was far more complicated than a list of character flaws. For example, it was clear to us that multiple IT companies had misled the state about the readiness of their software. Months later, in fact, Maryland collected $45 million from its lead IT contractor.[31] But having failed to tell a reasonable story about responsibility, we were sitting ducks for shouldering all the blame.

Tell a Balanced Story

Rather than try to evade questions of responsibility, health officials can run right at them, accepting fault for some part of the problem, while being clear and detailed about the role of others as well. If done calmly, and with credibility, this approach spreads the blame around where it is due, reducing the risk that any one organization will unfairly bear full responsibility or feel unfairly accused.

Executing this maneuver is complicated. One way to proceed is by arranging for a review by a trusted group of experts and then accepting their judgment when the review is completed. As discussed in Chapter 9, the FDA used this approach when beset by allegations that a medical device had been allowed onto the market inappropriately. An internal report written by several senior FDA officials attributed shares of responsibility to individuals at the agency, to members of Congress, and to weak review policies. The report led to the implementation of many policy changes to prevent the situation from happening again.

Alternatively, agency leaders can just address the issue of responsibility themselves. This is what I chose to do during a difficult moment at the FDA, when I was serving as Principal Deputy Commissioner. In 2010, it was discovered that a pharmaceutical company had conducted a "phantom recall"—sending its own staff into pharmacies to buy back an entire lot of ibuprofen that was substandard rather than announcing a public recall. The actions bore a striking resemblance to the Mel Brooks comedy *High*

---

[31] Cohn M, McDaniels AK. Maryland to recoup $45 million it paid to rebuild failed health exchange. *The Baltimore Sun.* 21 June 2015.

Anxiety, in which a character proposes buying up all the newspapers to avoid bad press.[32]

When word of the phantom recall surfaced, members of Congress demanded answers and called a hearing to explore how the FDA could have possibly let it happen. I was the FDA's main witness.

One approach would have been to simply blame the company. After all, the company bore responsibility for the manufacturing problems and the ridiculous attempt to cover it up. But once I reviewed all the facts myself, I took a different approach.

> Regardless of the behavior of a company, it is FDA's job to do everything possible to protect the public. It was clear in November 2008 that the Motrin lots did not meet specifications. Yet the actual recall did not happen until early August of the following year. This took too long.[33]

The candid admission seemed to surprise some members of Congress, who responded with reasonable questions about what happened and what could be done to prevent the situation from happening again. The committee also reacted well to my explanation that the company's deception had in part thrown the agency off the scent of misbehavior. In fact, the news stories the next day reflected this more nuanced picture. For example, the Associated Press reported:

> Johnson & Johnson executives and the Food and Drug Administration both shouldered the blame yesterday for a secret recall in which hired contractors quietly bought up defective painkillers to clear them from store shelves.
>
> J&J's chief executive, William Weldon, told House lawmakers the company made a mistake in conducting the "phantom recall," which is one of a string of problems that have drawn congressional scrutiny.
>
> In the same committee hearing, the FDA's deputy commissioner, Dr. Joshua Sharfstein, said his agency should have acted sooner to halt J&J's plan. At the

---

[32] "The first thing I want you to do is get a truck. A big truck. Then you go around to all the newspaper . . . All the stands. You put the paper . . . Perhaps it's not a good idea." *High Anxiety.* Fox Studios, 1977.

[33] Sharfstein JM. Johnson and Johnson's recall of Children's Tylenol and other children's medicines and the phantom recall of Motrin (Part 2). Statement of Joshua M. Sharfstein, M.D., Principal Deputy Commissioner, U.S. Food and Drug Administration, Department of Health and Human Services, before the Committee on Oversight and Government Reform, U.S. House of Representatives. 30 September 2010. Accessed January 22, 2018, at https://oversight.house.gov/wp-content/uploads/2012/02/20100930Sharfstein.pdf .

same time, though, he stressed that regulators were not aware of the deceptive nature of the recall.[34]

Another health leader who took a balanced approach to responsibility in a similar situation was Dr. Lauren Smith, Interim Commissioner of the Massachusetts Department of Public Health in 2012. She testified in Congress about the outbreak of meningitis caused by unsterile conditions at a pharmacy compounding agency located in her state. Instead of just blaming the company, Dr. Smith did not spare any details in describing failures of oversight by the Massachusetts Board of Pharmacy, which was affiliated with the Health Department. The Board had backed off possible restrictions on the pharmacy, failed to take action based on knowledge of fraud, and missed opportunities to respond to warnings sent by officials in Colorado. She said that "troubling questions" remain about the actions of the Board and described initial steps including firing responsible officials, shutting down the implicated facility, suspending operations of affiliated companies, and issuing a series of emergency regulations.

"The Board of Pharmacy's prior approach . . . is no longer sufficient to keep pace with the changing nature of the industry," she testified. "I pledge to you that Massachusetts will do whatever we can, make any changes, and identify any areas of new law to make sure something like this never happens again. We intend to identify responsibility but also focus on reforms that will be effective and lasting."[35] It was a tough hearing, but even adversarial members of Congress like Rep. Morgan Griffith of Virginia said, "I appreciate your coming forward and saying mistakes were made."[36] He followed with a series of specific substantive questions that respected her continued credibility in addressing the crisis.

Several months into the caustic news coverage about Maryland's health insurance exchange, I had another chance to address the issue of responsibility. On April 2, 2014, I spent a marathon day testifying both in Congress and in the Maryland General Assembly about what had gone wrong with our website's launch and what we intended to do next. I stated, "Maryland's

---

[34] Perrone M. J&J, FDA take blame for "phantom recall." Associated Press. 1 October 2010.

[35] Smith L. Testimony of Dr. Lauren Smith, Interim Commissioner of the Massachusetts Department of Public Health. Subcommittee on Oversight and Investigations, House Committee on Energy and Commerce. 14 November 2012. Accessed June 11, 2017, at https://energycommerce.house. gov/sites/republicans.energycommerce.house.gov/files/Hearings/OI/20121114/HHRG-112-IF02-WState-SmithL-20121114.pdf.

[36] Fungal meningitis outbreak, government panel. C-Span. 14 November 2012.Accessed June 11, 2017, at https://www.c-span.org/video/?309397-3/fungal-meningitis-outbreak-government-panel&start=7029.

story includes decisions we wish we could make again, failures by multiple vendors, and too many IT frustrations to count."[37] The next day's *Washington Post* headline read, "Md. Health Official: Exchange Debacle Included 'Decisions We Wish We Could Make Again.'"

By acknowledging our errors, I created enough space to put forward what we were doing to fix the situation—and earn enough public support to get a second chance. It was far from an easy experience, but we survived with enough momentum to push forward with a different technology system. Defying all of the detractors who had assumed we were the gang that couldn't shoot straight, the second implementation worked well, and today Maryland has one of the most effective health insurance exchanges in the country.[38]

Conclusion

Arjen Boin and Paul 't Hart, scholars of crisis, have written, "Engaging in critical self-reflection amounts to political hara-kiri for today's policy makers."[39] Unfortunately, not engaging in critical self-reflection can be equally painful.

There are moments when every voice seems to advise against accepting responsibility. Agency staff do not want to endure adverse attention. Political leaders are loathe to give others partisan advantage. Lawyers point out that expressing remorse and apologizing might lead to legal liability.[40] Health officials themselves worry silently about embarrassment and humiliation.

As a result, it is the rare public official willing to step forward, say something went wrong, and commit to fixing it. Ironically, this reality may make apologizing easier to do so. These days, the bar is pretty low for candor from public officials. Taking at least some blame may not accomplish every goal, but it often exceeds expectations. Sometimes, leadership means having to say you are sorry.

---

[37] Johnson J. Md. health official: Exchange debacle included "decisions we wish we could make again." *The Washington Post*. 3 April 2014.

[38] McDaniels AK, Cohn M. Health registry signups begin: State exchange enrolls 834 in the first day; no glitches reported. *The Baltimore Sun*. 2 November 2015.

[39] Boin A, Hart P. Public leadership in times of crisis: Mission impossible? *Public Administration Review*. 2003;63(5):544–553: 548.

[40] Coombs WT. *Ongoing Crisis Communication: Planning, Managing and Responding*. 3rd ed. Los Angeles: SAGE, 2012: 27.

An important skill for leaders is to be able to receive criticism and shoulder responsibility without feeling it too intensely. Harsh statements in the media certainly sting. It is painful to think about loved ones reading insults and invective. But it is worth remembering that nobody is perfect, and it is impossible to make progress without failing from time to time. When faced with tough criticism, my own mantra during my most difficult days was from *The Godfather*: "It's not personal . . . it's strictly business."

And sometimes businesses fail. So there is one final taboo topic to mention: When to resign. In extreme situations, health officials sometimes conclude that it is necessary for them to accept all the blame, even beyond what is due, and step down in order for an agency to recover and move forward. This maneuver is known as "falling on one's sword." In September 2012, for example, the highly respected Massachusetts Health Commissioner Jonathan Auerbach resigned in the wake of a state laboratory scandal not of his making. At the time of leaving his position, he said:

> It is with deep regret and with a sense of responsibility to uphold the high ideals Governor Patrick demands that I announce today my resignation as Commissioner of the Department of Public Health.
>
> It is clear that there was insufficient quality monitoring, reporting, and investigating on the part of supervisors and managers surrounding the former Department of Public Health drug lab . . . —and ultimately, as Commissioner, the buck stops with me.

At first glance, this difficult experience might be considered a worst-case scenario. But in the process of resigning, Auerbach received a multitude of compliments for his career and his sense of responsibility from the mayor of Boston, the governor of Massachusetts, and many others. He went on to take a significant leadership role at the Centers for Disease Control and Prevention and remains revered in the field of public health.

Of course, not every health official is guaranteed an outpouring of thanks upon resigning. There are no such guarantees in public service. At one meeting of state health officers, one of my colleagues said he felt like a toy in the movie *Toy Story*, with elected officials playing the role of the kids. He said sadly, "When they're done with us, they'll throw us away." His point was that even doing a great job is no protection against a bad outcome.

This is indeed true. On one hand, uncertainty and unpredictability make public health a great and exciting field. On the other hand, these same attributes of the job are not always kind to health officials. In the blame wars that result from crisis, there is only so much that any one person can control. And yet, there is something liberating in such a dismal assessment. No matter the future may hold, health officials should recognize that accepting responsibility strategically and fixing problems still have the advantage of being the right things to do.

11 | Opportunity in Crisis

T HE FIRST MONDAY OF EVERY month that I served as health commissioner in Baltimore, I chaired the city's child fatality review. This was a multi-agency meeting to discuss the details of the unexplained deaths of children in the city. It was the most excruciating hour of my month—and also the most important.

Around the table in a conference room at nearby Mercy Medical Center sat representatives from the Health Department, the Office of the Chief Medical Examiner for the State of Maryland, the Department of Social Services, the local prosecutor, the city's mental health and addiction agencies, and the state's Department of Juvenile Services. The Assistant Medical Examiner started each meeting by reviewing the autopsy findings in a tragic case. Each agency official had their pertinent records at the ready to inform the discussion.

As chair, I started by asking clarifying questions. Who was responsible for the baby when she was put to sleep face down in the bed, instead of on her back in a crib? Did someone in the school system try to intervene when a 7th grader became chronically absent and later dropped out to become involved in the illicit drug trade?

I eventually guided the discussion to specific ideas for how a death might have been prevented. For example:

- We reviewed the case of a baby who had died at the hands of a parent who had previously lost custody of her other children due to abuse. In our discussion, an official from the Department of Social Services asked whether it might be possible to know immediately which newborns were born to parents with such a worrisome record, so that the home's safety could be evaluated. She noted that a proposal to require an automatic "match" of social services records against birth records had failed a few years earlier in the Maryland General Assembly.

- Our review of multiple deaths of young infants in unsafe sleeping arrangements led to a conversation about ways to influence how parents put their kids to sleep in Baltimore. One Health Department worker proposed a citywide public health campaign encouraging safe sleep.
- We noticed that virtually all the teenagers murdered in Baltimore had thick files with the Department of Social Services and Department of Juvenile Services. This observation led to an effort of analyzing data to understand the trajectory of at risk youth in Baltimore.[1] The analysis revealed that homicide frequently followed many years of warning signs, including multiple arrests and trouble in school. Someone from the Department of Juvenile Services asked how it might be possible to enhance services for these youth at earlier ages.

After each child fatality review meeting, I walked several long blocks alone back to the Health Department, emotionally exhausted and deep in thought about how these ideas could be brought to reality. The child fatality review meeting was highly confidential, the discussions protected by a state law modeled on medical review committees; there was little chance of the discussion leaking out to the public. So there were no inquiring journalists or engaged legislators—at least, not yet.

That is, I recognized that real progress in these areas might well require media attention and legislative action. Somehow, we had to impart urgency and importance to the various ideas that had emerged. We had to create deadlines for action, a sense that something needed to be done.

In short, we had to awaken a sense of crisis.

In general, crisis management is a reactive skill. Health officials are confronted with a daily barrage of stressors, some of which require a full-scale response. But health officials can also use the language and urgency of crisis to promote action on real concerns that otherwise might slip below the radar.

Some consider this a radical idea. The job of a health official, in their mind, is to methodically develop an agenda based on evidence and let the

---

[1] Office of Epidemiology and Planning and Office of Youth Violence Prevention, Baltimore City Health Department. Examination of Youth Violence in Baltimore, 2002–2007. August 2009. Available online at http://baltimorehealth.org/wp-content/uploads/2016/06/Examination-of-Youth-Violence-in-Baltimore-City-FINAL.pdf.

political tides ebb and flow around them. According to this view, ginning up a crisis is unseemly and dangerous and likely to involve playing too closely to the highly charged third rail of politics.

My view is informed by the following statement:. The nature of public health makes it difficult, if not impossible, to draw attention to critical policy issues solely by strategic planning. Public health has no burning buildings, no sirens, and no heroic surgeries. Our ideas frequently draw the ire of entrenched interests opposed to safety measures. Many of those whose health we are seeking to advance have little political capital of their own. Yet the history of public health is replete with examples of the impossible becoming possible only during crisis. Health officials who are afraid to arouse a sense of crisis—when there is ample justification—are potentially squandering one of their most important tools for change. The third rail, after all, is where the power is.

That's why the Baltimore City Health Department used the findings of the child fatality review to focus the media and the public on the urgent need for prevention—and then took advantage of the attention to advocate for legislation and resources. For example:

- Citing the case of the parents with histories of abuse who killed yet another child, we fought successfully for the passage of a "birth match" bill in Maryland that is now considered a national model.[2]
- Calling attention to the dozens of babies who died in unsafe sleep conditions, we launched a citywide effort known as B'More for Healthy Babies. We raised funds from our state's leading insurer and others to support a communications campaign. Created by the Center for Communication Programs at the Johns Hopkins Bloomberg School of Public Health, the campaign featured interviews with parents who had lost their children in unsafe sleeping arrangements (Figure 11.1).[3] The city then showed these videos in jury waiting areas, social service departments, and on television. Along with other important strategies, this effort contributed to a dramatic fall in

---

[2] Shaw TV, Barth RP, Mattingly J, Ayer D, Berry S. Child welfare birth match: Timely use of child welfare administrative data to protect newborns. *Journal of Public Child Welfare* 2013;7(2):217–234.
[3] Johns Hopkins Center for Communications Programs. USA Maternal/Child Health: B'More Babies Safe Sleep Campaign Video. 3 March 2011. Accessed June 22, 2017, at https://www.youtube.com/watch?v=yBBiG6e4xRw&t=188s.

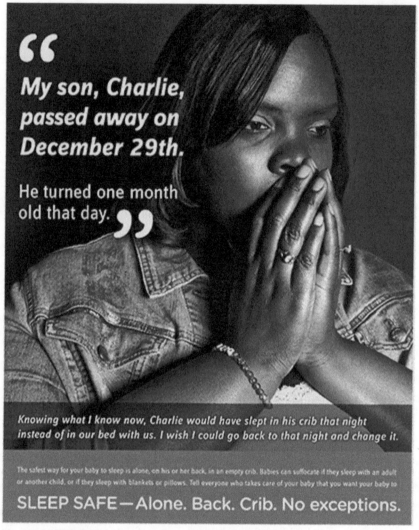

Inside the poster:

> **"**
> *My son, Charlie, passed away on December 29th.*
>
> He turned one month old that day. **"**
>
> *Knowing what I know now, Charlie would have slept in his crib that night instead of in our bed with us. I wish I could go back to that night and change it.*
>
> The safest way for your baby to sleep is alone, on his or her back, in an empty crib. Babies can suffocate if they sleep with an adult or another child, or if they sleep with blankets or pillows. Tell everyone who takes care of your baby that you want your baby to
>
> SLEEP SAFE—Alone. Back. Crib. No exceptions.

FIGURE 11.1 Campaign poster for B'More for Healthy Babies

unsafe sleep-related deaths and the lowest city infant mortality rate on record.[4]

- Pointing to our analysis based on child fatality review data, we described violence among adolescents as a public health crisis and raised substantial private funds for anti-violence programs based on

---

[4] Baltimore City Health Department. Baltimore city experiences record low infant mortality rate in 2015. 5 October 2016. Available online at http://health.baltimorecity.gov/news/press-releases/2016-10-05-baltimore-city-experiences-record-low-infant-mortality-rate-2015.

public health principles, which aimed both to deter retaliation and to provide essential social support. The projects were found to lessen attitudes likely to lead to violence, including the perception that guns were needed to settle disputes. And they reduced the number of shootings.[5]

How to arouse a sense of crisis? There is no single recipe. Public health officials should have at the ready the ability to frame a situation as an urgent matter in need of attention, a plan to take short-term action, and a commitment to seeking lasting policy change.

Framing a Problem

There's a lot more to crises than the word "crisis." That's because a crisis is not defined by language; it's a social understanding about a threat. It's a shared feeling of urgency. Generating this understanding is particularly challenging when others have reasons to disagree with the underlying facts, dismiss the importance of the problem, and reject proposed solutions. That's why health leader should aim first to create the right context for the issue before using the word "crisis."

Otherwise, health officials may feel like they are shouting fire in a theater while everyone keeps watching the movie. Exhibit A: Oysters. In fall of 2009, senior FDA officials reviewed the data on the risks involved with eating raw Gulf Coast oysters sold in the summer. These oysters are often contaminated with *Vibrio vulnificus*, a bacteria that can cause a horrible sepsis and death. In fact, a common story is someone with diabetes or mild liver dysfunction who has a few raw oysters and dies several days later.[6] I even recall a story of someone dying from this hideous infection on his honeymoon.

In October 2009, a senior agency official flew to a national meeting of seafood officials 2009 and told them *Vibrio vulnificus* infections posed a serious health threat—a cisis—that required an immediate fix. He announced that the FDA would soon be requiring a remediation step, such as pressure treating the oysters to kill the bacteria, before raw Gulf Coast

---

[5] Webster DW, Whitehill, JM, Vernick JS, Parker EM. Evaluation of Baltimore's Safe Streets program: Effects on attitudes, participants' experiences, and gun violence. 11 January 2012. Accessed June 22, 2017, at http://www.jhsph.edu/research/centers-and-institutes/center-for-prevention-of-youth-violence/field_reports/2012_01_11.Executive%20SummaryofSafeStreetsEval.pdf.
[6] Kestin S. The Gulf's deadly harvest. *South Florida Sun-Sentinel*. 14 September 2016.

oysters could be sold in the summertime. He expected the seafood industry would understand the need for prompt action to save lives.

The response was immediate: total opposition. Gulf state seafood officials argued that the danger had been known for years, that there was no reason to change practice now, and that safety measures would have devastating economic consequences. The news reports that followed focused on the economic, rather than the public health, side of the story. For example, on October 28, 2009, the front page of the *Times Picayune* read:

> At the small warehouse tucked away in the back side of the French Quarter, the shuckers at P&J Oyster Co. have arrived before daybreak for 133 years. Their in-shell and shucked oysters have been on the menus of generations of restaurateurs, from oysters on the halfshell at Acme Oyster House and Casemento's to the seafood gumbo at Dickie Brennan's Steakhouse. In less than two years, the tradition could become obsolete for seven months out of the year, based on newly announced oyster guidelines from the Food and Drug Administration.[7]

I was the FDA official sent to explain what was happening to two irate members of the Louisiana Congressional delegation at a meeting in the US Capitol. I attempted to test the idea that "at least we can agree no one should die from eating an oyster on his or her honeymoon." One of the Congressman responded, "What about chicken salad, doctor? Doesn't chicken salad kill more people?" The meeting went downhill from there. As a member of the US Senate and a member of the US House of Representatives took turns berating me and the agency, I thought about the path not traveled.

It's possible that the political realities would have made any progress on *Vibrio vulnificus* impossible. But it is worth imagining what might have happened had the FDA started not by announcing a new policy but rather by working to define the issue publicly as an urgent health concern. The FDA could have published a public notice asking for input about the health risks of raw Gulf Coast oysters in the summer or could have developed an analysis about preventable deaths from various foods, including raw Gulf Coast oysters. The agency could have drawn attention to California, which had earlier adopted a policy of not selling raw Gulf Coast oysters in the summer a few years earlier and had saved lives. This approach would have

---

[7] Kirkham C. Louisiana blasts new FDA rule requiring oysters to be sterilized to prevent rare bacterial illness. *New Orleans Times Picayune.* 28 October 2009.

had the effect of highlighting important data and stories before the agency made decisions about what to do next.

But now it was too late. Without public understanding or administration support, the FDA retracted the policy. Seven years later, it has yet to be implemented. Congress even set up new barriers to the FDA taking action.[8]

A few months later, the agency took a different approach on a different issue: the health risks of caffeinated alcoholic beverages. Instead of declaring a crisis and announcing immediate action, our first step was to elevate the issue and call for more information to inform a regulatory approach. "The FDA is not aware of any basis that manufacturers have to conclude that the use of caffeine added to alcoholic beverages is generally recognized as safe," I said.[9] This information request led reporters to seek out experts, who explained that these products combined high levels of alcohol with high levels of caffeine and induced a state that some called "wide awake drunk."

The experts—and not, in the first instance, our agency—explained the evidence that the consumption of caffeinated alcoholic beverages was associated with motor vehicle accidents, sexual assaults, and alcohol poisoning.[10] The ensuing coverage focused attention on these harms and set the frame as a public health crisis first and a regulatory issue second. A few months later, few were surprised (and even fewer objected) when the FDA moved to remove these products from the market.[11]

The Role of Research

The FDA's success with caffeinated alcoholic beverages, reflects, in part, how data and research can support the recognition of a problem as an urgent matter requiring attention. Collaboration between academic experts and public health officials can pay tremendous dividends in moving a problem from "longstanding" to "pressing."

For example, a new study might provide updated information on the scale of an issue; a quick expression of surprise and concern by public

[8] Kestin S. The Gulf's deadly harvest. *South Florida Sun-Sentinel.* 14 September 2016.

[9] Harris G. FDA says it may ban alcoholic drinks with caffeine. The New York Times. 13 November 2009.

[10] Zajac A. FDA to examine safety of caffeinated alcoholic beverages. *The Los Angeles Times.* 13 November 2009.

[11] Goodnough A. Caffeine illegal in alcohol, FDA warns 4 beverage-makers. *The New York Times.* 18 November 2010.

health officials can begin to build a sense of crisis. A scientific publication might prove that there are new opportunities for prevention or intervention; health officials can respond with urgency to implement the findings.

It helps to have researchers willing to engage with policymakers and, where possible, ready to come forward to testify to the need for action in the short term. For their part, health officials should recognize that research exposing problems may not just create a public relations headache but may also provide an opportunity to seize the moment.

Taking Action

As the public begins to understand that a problem is an urgent health challenge, the agency can itself act with purpose, even if its options are limited. Nothing reinforces a sense of crisis like an agency behaving like there is a crisis.

For example, in 2006, when a major heat wave loomed at the start of a summer in Baltimore, the Health Department could have quietly prepared a budget proposal for resources to protect vulnerable city residents. Instead, we announced a "code red heat alert" and launched a plan to open cooling centers and restrict certain outside activities.[12] We knew these steps would only directly help a small fraction of the population. But actually taking action, however small, reinforced our overall message of caution and led others to contribute to the effort. Reporters also had a better sense of the severity of the situation, and this increased the chance that members of the public would pay attention and take steps to protect themselves. We eventually did receive extra local and state resources to support the plan.

There are many steps that underfunded agencies can take to express urgency. Health officials can activate their incident command system (see Chapter 7), create a novel surveillance report, hold a public hearing, set up a special clinic, or launch outreach programs on social media. Each step deepens public understanding that there is really a need for focused attention and action.

Simple and direct actions can run alongside and reinforce broader policy initiatives. An example can be found in how Maryland's Health Department took on the issue of crib bumper pads. In 2011, medical

---

[12] Martin JL. Responding to the effects of extreme heat: Baltimore city's code red program. *Health Security.* 2016 Apr;14(2):71–77.

journal articles[13] and news reports raised awareness that these products, which parents buy for decoration and to soften the inside of the crib slats, can cause suffocation and strangulation.[14] In response, the Health Department called for public comment about the safety of these products and appointed an advisory committee to review the public comments and make recommendations. The committee urged attention to the risks of crib bumper pads and urged the state to ban their sale. As *The Baltimore Sun* reported, "Maryland could become the first state in the nation to ban the sale of bumper pads that line the inside of cribs after a state panel recommended Friday that health officials declare them a hazard because they can suffocate or strangle babies."[15] And the newspaper soon added an editorial calling on the state to move forward with a ban.[16]

Several weeks later, the Health Department did propose a regulation to ban the sale of crib bumper pads in Maryland. Significantly, the Health Department wrapped this proposal in a strong public health warning about their use. At a press event announcing the proposal, leading pediatricians and outreach workers provided a clear and consistent message to parents. As secretary of health at the time, I was quoted as saying, "The ABCs of safe sleep. Babies should sleep Alone, on their Backs, in the Crib—along with a 'D.' Don't use a bumper."[17] This message was both good public health practice and a clear signal of the need for policy change.

Manufacturers of crib bumper pads resisted the idea of a ban, hiring lobbyists and aiming to get the state's General Assembly to block the regulation. But the Health Department had framed the issue as a matter of infant safety and demonstrated its resolve through effective public messaging. After making a few changes in response to issues raised in the public comment period, the Health Department finalized the ban, which took effect on June 21, 2013.

---

[13] Thach BT, Rutherford GW Jr, Harris K. Deaths and injuries attributed to infant crib bumper pads. *Journal of Pediatrics*. 2007 Sep;151(3):271–274, 274.e1–3.

[14] Gabler L. Agency fails to probe deaths linked to popular baby products. *The Chicago Tribune*. 29 March 2011.

[15] Walker A. Maryland task force recommends banning crib bumpers. *The Baltimore Sun*. 20 May 2011.

[16] Time to ban bumpers. *The Baltimore Sun*. 24 May 2011.

[17] Fujii A. Md. health officials seek ban on crib bumper pads. CBS Baltimore. 27 September 2011. Accessed June 22, 2017, at http://baltimore.cbslocal.com/2011/09/27/md-officials-to-announce-steps-on-baby-crib-pads-2/.

Working for Change

The third step for health agencies to establish the sense of a crisis is by directly and powerfully advocating for meaningful solutions. Absent this step, just describing a problem may simply increase public anxiety, and modest responses may promote a cynical perception that nothing serious will happen. At the right moment, calling for bold action forces the public and policymakers to stop and pay attention.

I learned this lesson in an unexpected way through a response to a case from child fatality review.

The basic details: Two Baltimore parents had brought their young infant with a fever and symptoms of an upper respiratory infection to an emergency department in the city. Nothing unusual. The hospital team provided all the recommended care: hydration, blood work, and antibiotics. There were no warning signs that anything was amiss. Several hours later, however, the child returned to the emergency department in cardiopulmonary arrest and died.

The autopsy revealed the cause of death to be an inadvertent overdose of over-the-counter cough and cold medications, which both the parents and grandparents had been giving without telling one another. Further review found that four children had died under similar circumstances over the previous several years. I recalled from my training in pediatrics that these products had never been proven effective in clinical trials. And so, together with a senior pediatrician at Johns Hopkins,[18] we called all the chairs of pediatric departments in the city and asked whether they would sign a statement urging parents never to give these products to young children. Without exception, they agreed.

Our announcement was a public health success. "Parents warned on cold remedies," read the front-page headline of *The Baltimore Sun*.[19] One of our co-signers, the head of the local chapter of the American Academy of Pediatrics, wound up on a national daytime talk show explaining our advice.[20]

Soon after, however, the excitement faded—and so did the sense of urgency. I resigned myself to the idea that we would not be able to get people to pay attention to the risks of over-the-counter cough and cold medications for more than a few days. Then, fortunately, a neighbor in

---

[18] The fantastic Dr. Janet Serwint.
[19] Bor J. Parents warned on cold remedies. *The Baltimore Sun*. 27 October 2006.
[20] The incomparable Dr. Daniel J. Levy.

Baltimore emailed me with a simple question: If these products carry serious risks and have never been shown to have benefits, why are they still being sold?

I asked a medical student[21] spending time at the Health Department to review this question, and she reported back that the products had made it onto the market through a poorly understood mechanism called the monograph process. Under this process, products must be "generally recognized as safe and effective" to be sold. Yet for pediatric cough and cold medications, there was no convincing data to support either safety or effectiveness, and the pediatric community "generally recognized" the products as unsafe and ineffective. We decided that enough was enough: Together with a group of experts, we petitioned the FDA to take these products off the market for young children altogether.

We did not expect to see results quickly. But the combination of a clear health framing, urgency represented by our warning to the public, and our advocating for major change convinced reporter Gardiner Harris at *The New York Times*, and his editors, to give the issue space on page 1.[22] I found myself interviewed on multiple national television networks and quoted in many newspapers and magazines.[23] The enormous publicity led the FDA to call for an advisory committee meeting on the safety of these products, and when the dust settled, the manufacturers voluntarily removed these products for children under age four from the national market. Subsequent research has documented that this action led to large declines in poison control calls and emergency department visits.[24]

In retrospect, we couldn't have planned it any better even if we had tried. Had the Health Department called for a ban before releasing information on the problem, nobody would have understood what we were doing. Our citywide alert had the effect of demonstrating commitment and urgency. Then, by calling publicly for decisive action, we supported the ability of the FDA and manufacturers to do what was needed to save lives.

---

[21] The brilliant Marisa North of the Johns Hopkins School of Medicine.

[22] Harris G. U.S. reviewing safety of children's cough drugs. *The New York Times*. 2 March 2007.

[23] Much to the delight of many in city government, I was even invited on the Tyra Banks Show, led by the famous model. However, after sending in a photo of myself to the producer as requested, I was told they were "taking the show in a different direction." Former Mayor Sheila Dixon still reminds me about this snub.

[24] See, e.g., Mazer-Amirshahi M, Reid N, van den Anker J, Litovitz T. Effect of cough and cold medication restriction and label changes on pediatric ingestions reported to United States poison centers. *Journal of Pediatrics*. 2013 Nov;163(5):1372–1376. Shehab N, Schaefer MK, Kegler SR, Budnitz DS. Adverse events from cough and cold medications after a market withdrawal of products labeled for infants. *Pediatrics*. 2010 Dec;126(6):1100–1107.

Too Many Crises?

In April 2017, dean of the Boston University School of Public Health Dr. Sandro Galea wrote a note to his students and faculty called "Crying crisis." He called for people in the field of public health to distinguish between "the immediate and the important" and reserve the use of the word "crisis" for situations that "affect large numbers of people," "threaten health over the long term," and "require the adoption of large scale solutions." Galea cited climate change as an example of a genuine crisis for public health.[25]

Similarly, in *The New England Journal of Medicine*, Rebecca Haffajee, Wendy Parmet, and Michelle Mello expressed caution about the use of emergency declarations for "garden variety health threats." They write:

> If this crucial tool is used too readily, public health officials may find themselves like the boy who cried wolf: their warnings about emergencies may go unheeded. Moreover, the public may lose trust in health officials, which may result in a loss of political legitimacy as well as a backlash against public health laws more generally.[26]

I agree with these experts that it is inadvisable for health officials to treat every potential threat or daily disturbance as a crisis, exhausting staff and undermining the capacity of the agency to do its regular work. Yet I disagree with the idea that the best way to use the power of crisis is rarely and only when as much as possible is at stake.

My argument starts with the point that there are many issues beyond national or global calamities that matter a great deal to a great many people. What is one person's "garden variety" health threat is another person's life or death situation. For example, as I am writing these words, *The New York Times* is reporting that British regulations that permitted the use of flammable materials to wrap buildings contributed to the horrific inferno that killed more than 75 Londoners.[27] I can imagine that, months ago, an enterprising health official might have tried to raise awareness of the risk of a catastrophic fire to generate public demand for higher safety standards.

<hr/>

[25] Galea S. Crying crisis. 23 April 2017. Accessed June 22, 2017, at https://www.bu.edu/sph/2017/04/23/crying-crisis/.
[26] Haffajee R, Parmet WE, Mello MM. What is a public health "emergency"? *The New England Journal of Medicine.* 2014 Sep 11;371(11):986–988.
[27] Kirkpatrick DD. Hakim D, Glanzjune. Why Grenfell Tower burned: Regulators put cost before safety. *The New York Times.* 24 June 2017.

The official might have even used the word "crisis," as in, "This is a crisis waiting to happen." Such a campaign might have broken the proposed rule of reserving the term "crisis" to issues involving hundreds of thousands or millions of people. It might also have helped to avert a terrible tragedy.

To paraphrase former House Speaker Tip O'Neill, all public health crises are local. The public cares deeply about risks to their own health and the health of their communities. Urgent threats to their well-being are, indeed, crises. Health officials who use the word and the concept wisely are doing their jobs. By contrast, a Health Department that responds cautiously to local challenges and decides against extraordinary action just because only a few lives are on the line does not win points for safeguarding the use of the term "crisis." Rather, the agency risks making itself irrelevant.

The goal of smart and purposeful use of the tools of crisis leadership and management is not to overuse the term or to cry wolf. Rather the goal is to help the public recognize that there is, in fact, an urgent matter that demands action. The reward is not publicity; it is progress and trust. Moreover, by aggressively tackling the local issues that matter to communities, health officials gain the credibility needed to tackle larger and larger questions. They can link local challenges to the bigger picture, can building up awareness of national or global problems.

Certainly, there are traps to be avoided. One is the idea that just because someone else has declared a crisis, a health official must necessarily agree. Another trap is that believing that using the word "crisis" or declaring an emergency can ever stand alone. Calling a situation a crisis but doing little to address it reflects an inability to do the hard work of developing a case, taking steps that demonstrate urgency, and outlining responsible policy solutions. In 2017, for example, multiple state governors declared emergencies over opioid overdoses. One governor said the declaration emphasized the need for an "all hands on deck approach."[28] Another governor said, "It's time to call this what it is—an emergency."[29] But then what? The states had little in the way of real action to announce. Without a compelling plan, there is a risk that the public will eventually come to wonder whether these emergency declarations were primarily for the purpose of public relations.[30]

---

[28] Turque B. Maryland governor declares state of emergency for opioid crisis. *The Washington Post.* 1 March 2017.

[29] Leonard K. Arizona governor declares state of emergency over opioid crisis. *The Washington Examiner.* 5 June 2017.

[30] This risk exists for the federal government too. See Sharfstein J. The opioid emergency: Now what, Mr. President? *USA Today.* 25 August 2017.

In my mind, there is no number of well-managed crises that is too many. That's because the public recognizes the need to address genuine threats to health and well-being. On the other hand, poor leadership and management can lead to questions about "crying wolf" after just one use of the term "crisis." There are no shortcuts. Leading through crisis effectively requires an enormous commitment of time and energy It requires health officials who are strategic, ready, and able to use available administrative, legal, and rhetorical tools when the time is right.

Embracing Crisis

Crises occur so regularly that it should be a job requirement for health officials to be effective in recognizing them early and managing their response. But what about the further ability to pivot in a crisis to fight for long-term change, or the additional skill of awakening a sense of crisis to address a longstanding need?

These characteristics in managers and leaders are rarely sought, and even more rarely celebrated. That's because most people see crises more as challenges than as opportunities. The reluctance to embrace crisis is understandable. After all, trying and failing to squeeze opportunity from a crisis can embarrass or distract an agency and set back the careers of public officials.

So why risk it? Having experienced both the highs and the lows of leadership and management in crisis, I have my own answer to this question. The long version can be found in the pages of this book. The short version begins with the understanding that the skills to engage with crises can be studied, practiced, and improved over time. The task may be daunting, but it is hardly impossible.

It continues with the realization that addressing crises is as central to the history of public health as any other aspect of our field. Had officials in the past shied away from leadership in crisis, we would not have as safe food or as safe and as effective medications as we have today. The public expects that public health agencies will do what is necessary and sensible to save lives at the moments that really matter.

And it ends with the truth that there is so much more to be done.

Supplementary Materials: A Closer Look

APPENDIX 1 | In Depth: AIDS Activists and the FDA

MARK HARRINGTON

In 1987, the AIDS epidemic was seven years old and raging out of control. Hundreds of thousands of Americans already infected would die from the disease. By early 1988, 64,847 Americans had developed AIDS and 37,426 had died from it.[1]

Founded in 1987, the AIDS Coalition to Unleash Power, or ACT UP, represented a new, community-based, nonviolent direct-action movement directed at forcing government and other institutions to step up their efforts against the disease. ACT UP took on some of society's most powerful and conservative institutions, including the U.S. Food and Drug Administration (FDA). Within five years, ACT UP had FDA—among others—making radical policy transformations. Activists and people with AIDS developed unprecedented expertise, access, and power within biomedical research. We spurred the expedited release and broadened availability of treatments which increased the survival time of people newly diagnosed with HIV to levels near those not infected and drove the AIDS mortality rate down by more than 70%.

AIDS treatment activists created a new culture of information, empowerment, and collective support. They took on the US biomedical research establishment and wrought radical changes in research, drug approval, and empowerment of people with HIV. These transformations hold great promise for people at risk for life-threatening diseases—everybody, that is. In the long run, this can only make research more relevant and useful to people in their everyday lives. It offers the promise of speeding the discovery and distribution of therapies which will lengthen and improve the lives of people with life-threatening diseases.

ACT UP's first national demonstration, "Seize Control of the FDA," on October 11, 1988, kicked off an epic campaign to transform the drug testing system in the United States, a campaign that produced results far beyond its wildest dreams. AIDS activists forced the FDA, the National Institutes of Health (NIH), and drug companies to speed

---

[1] Centers for Disease Control, *HIV/AIDS Surveillance Report*, 1988.

up research and broaden access and provide new treatments which prolonged the lives of people with AIDS and prevented many opportunistic diseases.

Between 1988 and 1992, in response to demands by AIDS activists, the FDA developed a whole range of programs that would speed access to experimental therapies to people with life-threatening diseases, expand access outside of controlled clinical trials through Parallel Track, and approve drugs far earlier in the research process.

The FDA controlled all four routes for access to potential AIDS drugs. The FDA decided which drugs would be licensed and available *by prescription*. The FDA approved experimental treatments available *through clinical trials* at medical centers and in doctors' offices. The FDA could allow certain experimental drugs out on *special release programs* like Treatment IND or compassionate use. Finally, the FDA oversaw the *AIDS drug underground* and could allow or forbid PWA buyers' groups to import drugs approved abroad or to sell unlicensed substances to people with AIDS. The FDA could easily shut these organizations down, and sometimes threatened to.[2]

In March 1987, the FDA released new regulations which it claimed would provide access to experimental therapies to patients in extreme need while the drugs were still being tested. These regulations formalized a long-term policy of allowing single patients so-called "compassionate use" access to unapproved drugs. Under the new regulations, the FDA could designate a drug as Treatment IND (investigational new drug), and the drug company could then give it to people for whom approved therapies were not working.[3] The first AIDS drug released under Treatment IND was trimetrexate, an experimental treatment for *Pneumocystis* pneumonia, one of the most common AIDS-related opportunistic infections (OIs). The FDA would only allow trimetrexate for patients who could not tolerate the approved anti-PCP drugs, Bactrim and intravenous pentamidine. To receive trimetrexate, patients must have had "serious or life-threatening reactions" to *both* approved treatments. Patients without side effects from the other drugs, who were simply getting worse—patients with "refractory" PCP—were not allowed into the Treatment IND. So you could be dying of PCP, but if you didn't *have side effects from the drugs which weren't working anyway,* you couldn't get trimetrexate. It was a lethal bureaucratic catch-22.

By July 1988, only 89 patients had received trimetrexate through the Treatment IND, while thousands were dying of *Pneumocystis* pneumonia around the country. As the FDA caught wind of the impending October ACT UP demonstration, its negotiators changed their tune. On an August 5 meeting with activist attorneys, the FDA announced a change : they were going to rewrite the trimetrexate Treatment IND so that patients who were failing on approved drugs could get the drug.[4]

---

[2] In the 1970s, the U.S. Supreme Court held that the FDA could prevent people from importing laetrile, the putative anti-cancer drug, and could prosecute people for selling or buying laetrile; *U.S. v. Richardson*, 588 F. 2nd 1235 (9th Circuit, 1978), certiorari denied., 440 US 947 (1979), *rehearing denied*, 441 US 937 (1979).

[3] Title 21—Food and Drugs Chapter I—Food and Drug Administration. Department of Health and Human Services. Subchapter D—Drugs for Human Use. Part 312—Investigational New Drug Application. Subpart I—Expanded Access to Investigational Drugs for Treatment Use. https://www.accessdata.fda.gov/scripts/cdrh/cfdocs/cfcfr/CFRSearch.cfm?fr=312.300.

[4] Margaret McCarthy, transcript of FDA meeting, 5 August 1988.

The FDA could have done it all along. No new data had come in on trimetrexate. But community pressure had forced the FDA to change the way it interpreted its own rules. The rules were always arbitrary. Under existing law, the FDA could do as it saw fit. Now, activists were poised to change the FDA to do what was necessary to tackle the AIDS crisis.

Friday, October 7, 1988, hundreds of ACT UP members took buses down to Washington, D.C., to see the Names Project Quilt. Covering the entire Ellipse on the Mall, the portable cemetery commemorated the names of 8,288 people who had died of AIDS, a quarter of the national total to date. All day, speakers read aloud from the litany of names. People walked along canvas strips lining each block of six panels.

On October 11, 1988, ACT UP members from around the country made their way to the blocklike FDA building. Perhaps 1,500 activists surrounded the building. Groups from each city, and affinity groups from ACT UP/New York, clustered together in the street by the front entrance, before a double row of county cops. Each group had its own visual signature, signs, and themes; 176 activists were arrested.

The TV news coverage that evening was comprehensive and sympathetic. We were on all local stations, ABC, NBC, CBS, Fox, and CNN. Press coverage of the FDA demonstration was overwhelming. We made the front page in Boston, Baltimore, Dallas, Houston, Orlando, and Miami and were well-covered in Atlanta, Buffalo, Chicago, Detroit, Los Angeles, Memphis, New York, Philadelphia, San Francisco, St. Louis, Tampa, Tucson, and Washington, D.C. *USA Today* ran a story on the front page of its third section. The tone of the coverage was favorable. AIDS activism had gone national.

Among community newspapers, the coverage was euphoric. A turning point in the AIDS epidemic had been reached. In fighting for the rights of people with AIDS, some said, we were at the vanguard of a larger movement for patients' rights, a movement to revolutionize medical research for all diseases. As Robert Massa put it in New York's *Village Voice*,

> These activists seek nothing less than a revolution in medical research. They are challenging long-standing assumptions about drug development. For the demonstrators who gathered in Washington, what the researchers call good science is murder—especially in this epidemic, when experimental drugs may be a patient's last hope. ACT UP's critique rests on a single sentence that became a slogan of the FDA action: "A Drug Trial is Health Care Too."[5]

Kiki Mason, writing in the *New York Native*, was even more euphoric:

> In eighteen months, ACT UP and similar militant organizations across the country have turned the tide of AIDS activism and forever changed the traditional gay movement . . .
>
> If militant organizations maintain their pressure on the FDA, the process will move faster, and lives will be saved . . .

[5] Robert Massa, "Acting Up at the FDA: What AIDS Activists Want," *Village Voice*, 18 October 1988, p. 1.

In the long war on AIDS this past weekend may be remembered as Gettysburg. We still have much heartache and bloodshed ahead of us. We can take it. The tide has turned. Victory will be ours.[6]

The triumphal optimism unleashed by ACT UP at Seize Control of the FDA gave birth, over the next year, to a powerful, revolutionary, and, at first, almost utopian strain of treatment activism.

In 1989, ACT UP cracked the US research system wide open. The energies unleashed in 1987 and tested in a frenzied, scattershot approach throughout 1988 were about to be focused with single-minded intensity on the FDA-regulated, NIH-funded, pharmaceutical-dominated American drug testing system.

When the year opened, just one drug had been approved by the FDA to be sold for treating AIDS—AZT—and no drugs had been approved specifically to treat the AIDS-related opportunistic infections. After six months of relentless activist pressure, in June, the FDA approved the first two drugs for AIDS-related opportunistic infections, aerosolized pentamidine to prevent pneumonia (PCP) and DHPG (ganciclovir) for cytomegalovirus (CMV) retinitis, a viral disease which caused blindness.

In winter 1989, it seemed we might be able to make a strategic advance in our campaign for FDA reform. We needed a *cause célèbre* to expose the inadequacies of the present system—a clear, unambiguous example of a useful drug which was being withheld due to FDA restrictions. DHPG (ganciclovir), a drug to treat CMV retinitis in people with AIDS, was that drug.

In people with AIDS, CMV may invade the eyes, progressing rapidly to blindness and death, and can cause brain lesions, colitis, diarrhea, wasting, and pneumonia.

No drugs were approved for CMV. Researchers from two drug companies, Burroughs-Wellcome and Syntex, discovered DHPG (ganciclovir) in 1984. Neither one carried out controlled studies, since they were having a patent dispute over the drug. In the meantime, they distributed the drug to thousands of patients with CMV retinitis in the United States and Europe under a "compassionate use" program. By 1986, Syntex had won the patent battle. Rather than carry out careful studies, however, Syntex simply applied for FDA approval based on uncontrolled data from the distribution program.

In October 1987, following a harsh FDA review of the DHPG database, the FDA's Anti-Infective Drugs Advisory Committee rejected Syntex's application by a vote of 11 to 2, with the committee's two ophthalmologists the only dissenting voices.[7] In order to develop the missing efficacy data, the FDA, NIAID, and Syntex collaborated in late 1988 to introduce a package of clinical trials and expanded access programs. This package debuted to a nationwide furor on November 30, 1988.[8]

---

[6] Kiki Mason. "FDA: The Demo of the Year: With the Troops in Washington," *New York Native*, 24 October 1988, 13–17.

[7] Summary Minutes, 32nd meeting, FDA Anti-Infective Drugs Advisory Committee, 26–27 October 1987, pp. 6, 9. In October 1987, the FDA rejected the data as non-randomized, only partially-concurrent historically controlled. In June 1989, the FDA utilized the same dataset to approve the drug. In mid-1991, the FDA used far less impressive data from historical controls in approving ddI.

[8] See "HHS News" press release, U.S. Department of Health & Human Services, 30 November 1988; Gina Kolata, "Despite Promise in AIDS Cases, Drug Faces Testing Hurdle: FDA Restricts Access to Prevent Blindness," *The New York Times*, 13 December 1988; Marilyn Chase, "Drug for Blindness Linked to AIDS Is Kept Off Market Due to Miscues," *The Wall Street Journal*, 10 February 1989.

The FDA demanded comparative data from prospective, randomized studies, but doctors would not be willing to enroll their patients in a placebo-controlled study, for obvious reasons: CMV disease was sight-threatening and life-threatening, and there were no available alternatives. Before DHPG, patients with CMV used to go blind and die; after it was developed, they could maintain their eyesight for months or years.

So the FDA and NIAID developed a comparison of "immediate versus deferred" DHPG for CMV retinitis. They invented a new concept, that of "non-immediately sight-threatening CMV retinitis." Patients with non-immediately sight-threatening CMV retinitis would have to enroll in an AIDS Clinical Trials Group study (ACTG 071), in which they would be randomly assigned to receive DHPG immediately, or after 16 weeks or when disease progression occurred.

In the meantime, patients with immediately sight-threatening CMV retinitis could receive open-label DHPG through a Treatment IND, and those already receiving the drug would continue doing so under compassionate use.

Ophthalmologists and AIDS physicians felt that *all* cases of CMV retinitis were sight-threatening. The damage of CMV retinitis is irreversible. DHPG can only stop the growth of new viruses; the destruction of ocular tissue is permanent. Therefore, delayed treatment increased the risk of cumulative damage, including blindness and retinal detachment.

The invention of "non-immediately" sight-threatening CMV retinitis appeared to be a cruel scientific imposture created to justify a trial which appeared grossly unethical to most people with AIDS and their physicians. To us, this seemed to be a coercive maneuver to rapidly fill an unethical clinical trial by closing off other routes of access to DHPG.[9]

Physicians and activists disagreed. DHPG was already approved in four European countries.

Activists were enraged. ACT UP's Marty Robinson alerted *The New York Times*, which ran a series of articles about the controversy. Jim Eigo wrote that the DHPG protocols were "coercive, unnecessary, a waste of time and resources, unsafe and discriminatory."[10]

ACT UP zapped a February hearing on FDA regulation of AIDS and cancer drugs, where FDA Antiviral Division director Dr. Ellen Cooper recounted the story of the DHPG fiasco.[11]

[After the 1987 rejection of DHPG] we really felt . . . stuck between a rock and a hard place. On the one hand, we had a drug that had activity against the virus that caused these life- and sight-threatening infections and a strong belief among physicians that it worked. . . . But, on the other hand, we, at the FDA, are supposed to impartially review data and approve drugs based on clinical data that shows evidence of efficacy. And we had no objective data that was submitted in the NDA. . . . The real question . . . boils down to do we approve the

---

[9] The research establishment acknowledged its hypocrisy in an underhanded but revealing manner. Both the Treatment IND and the controlled ACTG 071 protocols had informed consent forms for the participants. The Treatment IND form informed participants that DHPG was believed to be 80% effective for treating CMV retinitis. The informed consent for the trial NIAID opened in November 1988, ACTG 071, omitted this fact. Nonetheless it enrolled just 18 subjects.

[10] Jim Eigo, "Blinded by Science: DHPG and the Conflict Between Clean Data and Humane Health Care," poster for V International Conference on AIDS, Montreal, June 1989.

[11] "DHPG Trials: A Monument to Regulatory Hypocrisy," ACT UP Fact Sheet, 1 February 1989.

drug based on the widely held belief, but not supported by the data in the NDA, or do we ask that a prospective collection of data from a controlled trial, in patients not at high risk of immediate blindness, be gathered, analyzed and submitted? We chose the latter, while still allowing widespread distribution of the drug to patients with immediately sight- or life-threatening infection.

If we had approved the drug on the basis of the widespread belief in the community . . . without the objective data, we feel that we would, indeed, be on treacherous grounds in defending that decision and, in fact, would be wide open to the charge of arbitrary decision making, although we certainly wouldn't be accused of being inflexible . . .

I have to say that the difference in the data between AZT and [DHPG] is the difference between night and day as far as the quality of that data . . .

[F]rom my point of view, FDA shares the blame for the inadequate development of the drug.[12]

A cohort of activists took the subway to the NIH campus to demand a meeting with NIAID Director Anthony Fauci. Much to their surprise, Fauci agreed to meet with them. They presented ACT UP's concerns about DHPG, demanded that the limits on access be removed, and asked Fauci to pressure the FDA to approve the drug.

Fauci agreed with ACT UP's demand that access to DHPG be restored to all who needed it and agreed to call FDA Commissioner Frank Young. He kept his promise to ACT UP, called him, and the FDA changed. Just five days after our demonstration, *The New York Times* documented a remarkably rapid shift by the NIH, one that heralded a break with FDA's position on DHPG: "Dr. Fauci called Dr. Young last Wednesday after a meeting with several representatives of the AIDS Coalition to Unleash Power . . . On Friday evening, Dr. Fauci called . . . a member of ACT UP, and told him that Dr. Young had agreed to meet with Dr. Fauci and other researchers to look again at ganciclovir data."[13] The tide began to turn.[14]

On March 2, 1989, Frank Young sent me a letter saying, "I have decided to reconvene our Anti-Infective Drugs Advisory Committee on May 2 to examine the latest data on the drug's safety and efficacy . . . Pending the May meeting, my staff has begun to work with Syntex Corporation to widen the availability of open label use of ganciclovir so that no patient with CMV Retinitis will be systematically excluded from receiving the drug."[15] NIAID put out a press release quoting Fauci saying that, "We have been increasingly convinced that this is the right thing to do, ethically and medically."[16] In other words, people

---

[12] Transcript, National Committee to Review Current Procedures for Approval of New Drugs for Cancer and AIDS [the Lasagna Committee], 1 February 1989, pp. 139–141.

[13] Gina Kolata, "FDA Said to Be Re-evaluating Order for More Studies on an AIDS Drug," *The New York Times*, 6 February 1989.

[14] Marilyn Chase, "Drug for Blindness Linked to AIDS Is Kept Off Market Due to Miscues," *The Wall Street Journal*, 10 February 1989.

[15] Frank E. Young, FDA Commissioner, letter to Mark Harrington, ACT UP/New York, 2 March 1989. See Gina Kolata, "FDA Approves the Use of an Experimental Drug for AIDS Patients' Eye Infections," *The New York Times*, 3 March 1989.

[16] NIAID AIDS Clinical Trials Alert, "Ganciclovir Access Assured for AIDS Patients with CMV Retinitis," 3 March 1989. Whereas Hoth delivered the news about the "state-of-the-art" trials of December, Fauci took credit for the turnaround of March.

who developed a new case of non-immediately sight-threatening CMV retinitis would no longer be forced to go onto the controlled trial of immediate versus deferred ganciclovir. Hundreds of people with AIDS would no longer have to risk blindness in order to provide definitive proof that ganciclovir worked.

With DHPG, ACT UP begun to reach out for allies *within* the scientific community—researchers from the NIH and primary physicians who treated AIDS patients. DHPG was a case study in how *not* to regulate AIDS drug development. Deficiencies in its trajectory helped show the way toward the Parallel Track.

In few diseases did patient advocates yet have full participatory powers in NIH-funded research, in FDA regulation, or in industry-sponsored trials.

By the end of 1990 ACT UP had achieved its goal of empowering people with HIV and their communities. People with HIV and activists from around the country would become members of all ACTG committees and sit as advisors on the FDA's Antiviral Drugs Advisory Committee. Drug companies routinely met with activists at earlier and earlier stages of drug development. The activist demand for participation and power in the research world led to major cultural changes in clinical research. Within a few years, cancer patients would develop new activist groups, inspired by ACT UP, to press more aggressively for better cancer research. Not only did ACT UP want full participation, it wanted to change the research agenda.

> We need equal resources given to research on anti-infectives [preventives and treatments for opportunistic infections] as well as to antiviral drugs. Treating or curing the major opportunistic infections must immediately become a priority.[17]

People of color, women, poor people, rural people, IV-drug users, prisoners, hemophiliacs, and children with HIV were routinely excluded from drug trials. AZT was still not approved in children, over two years after its approval in adults. Among adults, over 50% of AIDS patients could not tolerate AZT. They were effectively excluded from clinical research, since all trials studied AZT, required it, or compared a new treatment to it. We demanded that the quarantine of the under-represented populations, and of the AZT-intolerant, be ended.

> Trials must be designed for the real world: prophylaxis permitted, placebos banned, efficacy criteria flexible, and endpoints humane... As other drugs become recognized as prophylactic agents for various OIs, trial subjects must be permitted to use them.
>
> Our last demand is that a new, nationwide distribution program for promising experimental drugs for HIV and opportunistic infections, accessible to all without regard to income, must be established.[18]

---

[17] Transcript, "National Committee to Review Current Procedures for Approval of New Drugs for Cancer and AIDS," 2 May 1989.
[18] Transcript, "National Committee to Review Current Procedures for Approval of New Drugs for Cancer and AIDS," 2 May 1989.

ACT UP's Jim Eigo proposed a new system of "parallel trials." Jim had first conceived of this one year earlier. Now he fleshed it out, writing that

> ACT UP believes that it is the moral and legal responsibility of FDA, which is a consumer protection agency, to ensure the equal access of all immune suppressed people to experimental treatment where there is no alternative. . . . Whenever a drug trial *truly* requires a "homogeneous population," FDA, in the order to ensure equal access to promising treatment, should in the name of "justice" require that a drug sponsor conduct "*parallel trials*" with the different segments of the HIV-infected population that have been eliminated from the original trial.[19]

Jim's proposal was the seed of what soon became known as "Parallel Track." Within five months the first Parallel Track drug, didanosine (ddI), would be distributed to thousands of PWAs intolerant of AZT, while trials comparing ddI to AZT began.

Across town, an FDA advisory committee had just recommended approval for aerosolized pentamidine and DHPG. Two small, quick community-based trials had yielded a clear answer about aerosolized pentamidine where the government had failed to move quickly enough. ACT UP's Garry Kleinman testified to the FDA committee:

> We are here to tell you that AIDS activists will agitate relentlessly until there is a cure for AIDS. We will agitate until it becomes impossible for advisory committees, whose members appear to have no knowledge of nor sympathy for those people who live with AIDS daily to consign such drugs as DHPG to regulatory limbo. This is a war as real as any war. Give us the weapons so that we can defend ourselves."[20]

Later that month, the FDA approved DHPG without its ever having completed a single randomized, controlled clinical trial.[21] The DHPG case, like that of aerosolized pentamidine, was unusual, though in a different way. The drug was much more effective than most experimental AIDS therapies. It was analogous to penicillin—it caused the rapid resolution of a previously untreatable, rapidly fatal disease. DHPG could have been studied properly, in the mid-1980s, but by 1989, it was unfeasible and, many believed, unethical to do a controlled study. Yet such situations are quite rare. Most drugs are far less effective than DHPG, and hence the need for reliable controlled data is greater. The DHPG example made it look like randomized studies were unnecessary for proving efficacy, but DHPG was a unique case.[22]

The approval of aerosolized pentamidine and DHPG contributed to a new optimism about the prospects for rapidly controlling AIDS. After eight years of relentless pessimism, a few months of optimism were warranted. It fueled an explosive growth in AIDS treatment activism, providing momentum for numerous campaigns over the next few years.

---

[19] Jim Eigo, "Problems Between FDA and the Community," *AIDS Drugs Now*, p. 9.

[20] FDA Anti-Infective Drugs Advisory Committee, Volume II, 2 May 1989, pp. 204–205.

[21] See Bruce Ingersoll, "FDA Clears Syntex Drug, Ganciclovir, As Therapy for AIDS-Related Blindness," *The Wall Street Journal*, 27 June 1989; Gina Kolata, "FDA Gives Quick Approval [sic] To Two Drugs to Treat AIDS," *The New York Times*, 27 June 1989; Associated Press, "FDA Acts on AIDS Drugs," *New York Newsday*, 27 June 1989.

[22] DHPG fit four out of the five criteria for testing a drug without randomization as laid out by David P. Byar in "Design Considerations for AIDS Trials," *New England Journal of Medicine*, November 1990.

In summer 1989, ACT UP found itself with a national campaign on its hands to make ddI the first Parallel Track drug. The pieces and the players came together very fast. ACT UP held meetings with NIH's Fauci and FDA's Cooper in June. Later that month, Fauci endorsed Parallel Track after meeting with Project Inform in San Francisco. ACT UP/ New York met with Bristol-Myers, makers of ddI, in late June, and in July the company announced that it would put ddI out on Parallel Track. Congress held hearings, at which ACT UP's Jim Eigo testified. In August, ACT UP and Project Inform led a national coalition which persuaded an FDA advisory committee to endorse Parallel Track. The government named Jim Eigo and Martin Delaney to a committee writing up the Parallel Track regulations, and ddI began reaching thousands of PWAs in September.

Parallel Track emerged from the DHPG fiasco, the debates about fixing Treatment IND, and a year of treatment activism, from our confrontation at the FDA to the Lasagna committee to Montreal. It was a synthesis of ideas developed by activists, the FDA, and the NIH. Everyone agreed that the DHPG saga, where the drug had been given out on compassionate use while controlled trials were delayed until they were no longer feasible, was the wrong way to go. Also a mistake was the old-fashioned system of testing drugs in rigid, restrictive, slow studies and excluding anyone but the trial participants from access until the drugs had proved safe and effective. Parallel Track was to be a system of trials outside the formal controlled studies, open to people ineligible or unable to access the controlled studies, focusing on patients who had run out of treatment options. Parallel Track was intended to be far broader, easier to enroll in, and more inclusive than any Treatment IND program to date.

Each of the players had different interests in Parallel Track. The FDA hoped it would take the pressure off the approval process by providing access to selected patients at high risk of disease or death without other treatment options and unable to enroll in trials. The NIH hoped that it would make the patients who did enroll in the controlled trials likelier to stay in the study without lying or cheating. Drug companies willing to foot the expense thought it was a good means of building market share and physician and patient acceptability before approval and might be useful to obtain expedited approval. Treatment activists hoped that it might solve the problems of Treatment IND. People with AIDS thought it might provide them with access to experimental therapies which they wanted or believed would be helpful.

The truth was that people with HIV *might* benefit. The drug could, after all, do more harm than good, but that wouldn't be clear for years, after controlled studies were completed, if ever. In the meantime, everyone involved in Parallel Track was placing a giant bet. The bet was that the benefits of ddI would outweigh its risks in people for whom AZT was no longer working. If we were right, thousands of patients would benefit, possibly by having longer, healthier lives. If we were wrong, hundreds or thousands of people might get sick faster or die sooner.

It was a huge risk—but, in 1989, after the initial hopes and later disappointment engendered by AZT, many people with HIV were willing to take that risk. New therapeutic breakthroughs seemed to be coming so quickly that, it was felt, access to a new drug might prolong life long enough for "the cure" to emerge.[23]

---

[23] Martin Delaney, "Congressional Testimony, Presented on behalf of Project Inform and ACT UP San Francisco," 20 July 1989.

At the end of September 1989, the FDA approved the ddI Parallel Track program. Eight thousand people with AIDS enrolled in the first six months. Eventually, over 26,000 people with AIDS, for whom AZT was useless or toxic, would receive ddI from Bristol-Myers on Parallel Track. The regulations would eventually be released in May 1990.

Through the early and mid-1990s the FDA continued to respond to the evolving needs of people with AIDS, researches, and activists. In 1992, FDA Commissioner David Kessler promulgated new regulations formalizing the process by which ddI could be approved. The Accelerated Approval regulations provided that a drug could be approved based on surrogate marker data (such as CD4 changes—and later on, quantitative viral load) if the marker was reasonably likely to predict clinical benefit.[24] Drug manufacturers would have to promise to conduct post-marketing studies to prove their drugs actually provided clinical benefit. The promise of accelerated approval was clear—drugs which were safe and might be effective could be released sooner—but its downsides weren't as apparent. Long-term side effects may not have yet been observed at the time of approval. With its drug on the market, the sponsor had much less incentive to carry out promised post-marketing studies, and it would be impossible for the FDA to remove an approved drug unless it caused truly ghoulish side effects. Ultimately, then, Accelerated Approval, if the company didn't keep its end of the bargain, threatened to replace clear answers about how to use new drugs with rapid access in a vacuum of relevant information for doctors and patients.

The result, for people with HIV and their doctors, was a confusing and contradictory situation. People were being told that these new drugs were vital and life-saving, but there was no data that they, in fact, saved lives, and they were expensive, inconvenient, and toxic. The first drug released officially under accelerated approval was Hoffmann-LaRoche's ddC, a popular drug at the time because small surrogate marker studies suggested that ddC taken with AZT might be superior to AZT alone.

If the ddI experience hinted that accelerated approval might work, the ddC one showed that, in the hands of an opportunistic drug company, its requirements for post-marketing studies could easily be flouted.

In early 1993, incoming President Bill Clinton asked David Kessler to stay on as FDA commissioner. Kessler spent the next two years continuing to streamline and accelerate drug approval, particularly with AIDS drugs. Data from studies released later that year showed that the CD4 count surrogate marker did not actually predict clinical benefit with some anti-HIV drugs, such as ddC.

Together, activists, researchers, drug companies, and the FDA had rewritten the book on AIDS drug development. Now it was clear that some of our guesses had been wrong. Our interests as activists diverged from those of researchers and drug companies. Researchers were perfectly happy to monitor laboratory values and churn drugs out; industry was perfectly happy to license new drugs without ever showing that they extended health or life. People with HIV and their doctors, however, while still needing rapid access to new treatments, also needed answers about how best to use those new treatments. Drugs were being licensed more quickly than ever before. Once on the market, what

[24] FDA, "Accelerated Approval of New Drugs for Serious or Life-Threatening Diseases," *Federal Register* 57:239, 11 December 1992.

incentive did drug companies have to deepen our knowledge base about how to use them? Not as great an incentive as activists and people with HIV.

Treatment Action Group and other HIV treatment activists would begin to critically examine every activist dogma which had led to expedited access and accelerated approval of AIDS drugs. Within a year, some activists would be calling for larger, longer, more rigorous studies designed to prove clinical benefit, not just short-term CD4 T cell changes.

No one could have imagined that within three years a whole new class of anti-HIV drugs, the protease inhibitors, would have been developed, studied, and approved by the FDA. These drugs are more powerful than AZT and its cousins. Protease inhibitors can reduce HIV levels in the blood by 99% or more in some cases.

In February 1996, Abbott Laboratories announced that its protease inhibitor Ritonavir plus nucleoside analogues reduced the risk of death in people with advanced AIDS by 50% over six months. The drug was fully approved overnight by the FDA.

Once the drugs were approved and on the market, thousands of people with failing immune systems started to take them. Many people experienced drops in their HIV levels of 99% or more and corresponding CD4 T cell increases. Some people left the danger zone of low T cells and maintained healthy levels for many months. The full duration of the antiviral activity of the protease inhibitors is not yet known, since they are so new, but, thanks to treatment activism, more was learned about how to use them than was known about ddI, ddC, or d4T at the time of their accelerated approval. When used in combination with nucleoside analogues, the protease inhibitors provided the best control of HIV yet achieved.

By 2017, the FDA had approved over 40 drugs and fixed-dose combinations for sale in the United States to treat HIV-1 infection.[25] In addition the FDA has given "tentative approval" to 198 drugs and fixed-dose combination antiretrovirals for use in PEPFAR-supported country programs internationally.[26] Over 19 million people living with HIV around the world were receiving life-saving anti-HIV combination therapy. Seventeen million more were living with HIV but not yet on treatment, though all needed to be.

There still is no scalable cure or effective vaccine against HIV. But the crucible of the AIDS crisis showed how the FDA could respond, adapt, and become more flexible to adjust to a public health crisis, while not sacrificing the need for well-designed and informative clinical trials.

---

[25] FDA-Approved HIV Medicines. Last reviewed 17 August 2017. https://aidsinfo.nih.gov/understanding-hiv-aids/fact-sheets/21/58/fda-approved-hiv-medicines. A few antiretroviral drugs have been removed from the US market by their manufacturers, including ddC (zalcitabine; HIVID, from Roche) and saquinavir soft-gel capsules (Fortovase, Roche), both discontinued in 2006. The NNRTI delavirdine (Rescriptor, ViiV/GSK) will be discontinued in 2018.

[26] FDA. Approved and Tentatively Approved Antiretrovirals in Association with the President's Emergency Plan. Last updated 23 August 2017. https://www.fda.gov/InternationalPrograms/PEPFAR/ucm119231.htm.

APPENDIX 2 | Rethinking Science and Politics

REPRINTED FROM *The Millbank Quarterly* courtesy of the Millbank Memorial Fund.

Just as religions separate the sacred from the profane, many people separate science from politics. Science is a calling defined by the search for truth, using reproducible evidence, whereas politics is a vocation fully engaged in the messy circumstances and compromises of the real world. Such a binary divide suggests the importance of keeping politics out of science—in other words, letting experts define a policy to achieve an important health objective and then expecting that the political process will support and implement it.

This simple and seemingly persuasive framework, however, cannot overcome 3 major challenges in practice.

First, science often cannot determine whether there is enough evidence to justify a policy. In the fall of 2009, for example, the US Food and Drug Administration (FDA) began to examine the safety of a new type of food: caffeinated alcoholic beverages. From the outset, there was a clear basis for concern, as the products combined several beers' worth of alcohol with several colas' worth of caffeine, risking harm from a state of "wide-awake drunk." Added to this were credible reports of alcohol poisoning, assault, and motor vehicle accidents associated with the use of caffeinated alcoholic beverages by adolescents and young adults. Leading outside experts, including public health officials, called for the FDA to remove these products from the market. It was clear to many that the time to act was short while the market for these products was dominated by small and politically weak companies and before powerful, large alcohol manufacturers began to make these combination beverages themselves.

Inside the FDA, however, there was debate over whether there was enough evidence to make a definitive decision. Even though everyone had the same concerns, some scientists proposed waiting for a multiyear study of the biological effects of caffeine before taking action. Instead, in November 2010, the agency sent warning letters to the manufacturers, which led directly to the removal of these beverages from the market.[1] This move was certainly justified scientifically, but the actual decision to act was a judgment call supported by political appointees at the agency. Had the FDA followed the recommendations of its most cautious scientists, these risky products might still be widely available.

Second, some scientific and public health goals require political support and savvy to achieve. For example, about a decade ago, as health commissioner of Baltimore, I was faced with an increasing number of people experiencing homelessness who were dying in the cold of winter. As long as the problem was seen primarily as a health issue, we could not do much to help them. All our department could do was provide nursing and medical support and ask for assistance from other agencies and for communities to permit the opening of more shelters on cold nights.

But when the mayor jumped in to help, she did a lot more than support the health commissioner. She mobilized the housing authorities to provide emergency assistance and long-term vouchers, directed the police to increase patrols to support community shelters, and committed substantial resources to building a center to help people regain control over their lives.[2] In addition, she overcame the community's initial anger and frustration at meetings at which neighbors angrily opposed the temporary placement of an emergency shelter, telling them, as I recall, "I don't want people to die on the streets of my city."

Third, sometimes politicians' judgment may actually be better than scientists' judgment regarding the implementation of scientific and public health policies. Amid the panic over the possible spread of Ebola in the United States in 2014, a physician who had been exposed to Ebola in West Africa but who did not show any symptoms, returned home to our state. The state health department had to decide whether to quarantine him by force of law until the end of the 21-day incubation period.

We polled leading infectious disease experts both inside and outside the department. Some argued strongly in favor of a quarantine order, saying that it was the only way to gain public trust and that it was the only way we could establish a consistent policy over time. Others disagreed, saying that a quarantine order might send a message of distrust of health care workers, which in turn would fuel the fear of Ebola in the United States that was already spreading well beyond reason.

The governor resolved the question by asking the health department not to issue a quarantine order and instead to use the force of law only when it was really needed. Standing with our state's leading hospital systems at an extended press conference, the governor explained our state's approach far more clearly and persuasively than those of us at the health department ever could. As a result, we gained the public's trust without having to issue a quarantine order.[3]

Rather than keeping science and politics apart, we should seek the effective alignment and mutual respect of the practitioners of each craft. Scientific considerations can define the problem and propose solutions. Political skill and power can adapt the solutions to the environment and implement them effectively.

To be clear, this alignment does not mean that anything goes in the interplay of science and politics. Political agendas that misrepresent facts risk the public's health. It is not difficult to find examples of politicians distorting science in favor of political positions on such topics as climate change, marijuana policy, reproductive health care, and gun safety. In the face of evidence suggesting a policy will harm the public's health, politicians should acknowledge the cost of the policy and, if they still support it, defend it on other grounds. Frequently, however, politicians choose to deny or distort evidence, thereby undermining the public's understanding of the trade-offs at stake.

When community leaders wrongly insist that gun control measures have never been shown to reduce violence, the public is less able to appreciate the likely benefits of proposed policies. Similarly, when politicians misstate the evidence regarding the risks to adolescents of liberalizing marijuana laws, the public is impeded from fully understanding the potential drawbacks of change.

Yet it is precisely because this type of political distortion of scientific evidence is so common that we need to rethink the ideal relationship between science and politics. When politicians misrepresent data, scientists generally respond in the language of science. Although this may convince those judging the exchange as a debate, it rarely reverses the public's misunderstanding and confusion. A presidential candidate in a debate watched by 25 million people who states that children receive too many vaccines cannot be effectively countered by footnoted editorials in scientific journals. Instead, another political leader must stand up and not only provide the right evidence but also support the expertise of leading public health organizations.

Scientists most often become involved in politics in order to support candidates who support their points of view. A broader strategy on behalf of science is also needed. Such a strategy should offer support to politicians across the ideological spectrum who respect data and evidence and who support the alignment of politics and science. Engagement with politics is a wiser course than isolation. Some scientists will always believe that politics is a third rail that they should not touch and that should not touch them; over time, perhaps more will recognize that the third rail is where the power is.

References

1. US Food and Drug Administration. FDA warning letters issued to four makers of caffeinated alcoholic beverages: these beverages present a public health concern. November 17, 2010. http://www.fda.gov/NewsEvents/Newsroom/PressAnnouncements/ucm234109.htm. Accessed November 17, 2015.
2. Linskey A. Residents support city's homeless shelter plans. Baltimore Sun. February 2, 2009.
3. Sharfstein JM. On fear, distrust, and Ebola. JAMA. 2015;313:784. [PubMed]

APPENDIX 3 | Banishing "Stakeholders"

REPRINTED FROM *The Millbank Quarterly* courtesy of the Millbank Memorial Fund.
Every year since 1976, Lake Superior State University in Sault Ste. Marie, Michigan, has released a list of banished words—terms in the English language that deserve never to be spoken again. The university's 2016 list includes "stakeholder."[1] As one nominator put it, referring to the vampire fighter from *Dracula*, "Dr. Van Helsing should be the only stake holder."

In the world of health policy, stakeholders abound. The Centers for Disease Control and Prevention notes that stakeholders can be

- program managers and staff;
- local, state, and regional coalitions;
- advocacy partners;
- state education agencies, schools, and other educational groups;
- universities and educational institutions;
- local government, state legislators, and state governors;
- privately owned businesses and business associations;
- health care systems and the medical community;
- religious organizations;
- community organizations; and
- private citizens.[2]

Soon after this year's "banished words" list appeared, AcademyHealth convened a meeting "to bring together a diverse group of stakeholders to review and discuss policy priorities at the forefront of child health." The US Department of Health and Human Services then promoted the National Health IT Stakeholder Pledge and the National Stakeholder Strategy for Achieving Health Equity. The HealthCare Institute of New Jersey convened the New Jersey Healthcare Stakeholders Summit, and the California Department of Public Health published *The Stakeholder Brief.*

These organizations—and many, many more—use the term "stakeholder" to express the meaning of "one who is involved in or affected by a course of action," the third listed definition in Merriam-Webster's online dictionary (http://www.merriam-webster.com/

dictionary/stakeholder). An agency "reaches out to," "includes," "engages with," or otherwise "hears from" stakeholders to develop health policies that will work in the real world.

I understand the utility of a shorthand term to signify that policies are not being made in a bubble. But I stand with Lake Superior State University: The term "stakeholder" should be relegated to the same linguistic storage facility as "trepanation" and "orgone generator."

To start, "stakeholder" has a mercenary connotation. The original meaning of the term is a person who literally held the money of bettors while the game was on. This meaning evolved into a second definition: "a person, company, etc., with a concern or (esp. financial) interest in ensuring the success of an organization, business, system, etc."[3]

Such a word origin is especially curious when it comes to health policy because stakeholders, in fact, frequently do have financial interests in the issue at hand. Depending on the matter, "key stakeholders" may include hospitals, physician practices, pharmaceutical companies, long-term care facilities, managed care organizations, insurers, and health IT companies.

It is, of course, essential to listen to the perspectives of those whose bottom line is affected by regulation and policy, but a catchall phrase like "stakeholder" obscures the landscape in question, much like a dense fog. Consider the greater clarity achieved by changing the sentence "Medicare proposed cutting the reimbursement rate to $2,500 per procedure, but there is significant pushback from stakeholders" to "Medicare proposed cutting the reimbursement rate to $2,500 per procedure, but those whose rates would be cut are protesting."

As a business term, "stakeholder" carries an assumption that all stakes have equivalent intrinsic merit. There are strategies to "identify key stakeholders," books on and courses in "stakeholder management," and videos on how to "deal with angry stakeholders." A primary goal of this enterprise is to "make the stakeholders happy."

The purpose of good health policy, however, is not to make the stakeholders happy. Instead, the purpose is to advance the health of the public at reasonable cost. Sadly, a number of health regulations and payment policies include provisions that favor financially interested parties with negative or no benefit for the public at large. "Stakeholder engagement" can put such interested parties on the same level as the many individuals and families who pay more, suffer worse quality of care, or go without key preventive interventions. In essence, in a world where everyone is a "stakeholder," there is less room for the public interest.

Those who are skeptical of my concern over this terminology ought to attend a few more "stakeholder meetings." Many are filled with lobbyists whose job it is to restate established positions of industries or organizations, with little opportunity for give-and-take. Stakeholder meetings can last for hours and include dozens of people, some of whom have tussled and fought with one another for years.

A collection of "stakeholder meetings" is called a "stakeholder committee." Over many hours of debate and discussion, entrenched interests often take the opportunity to dig in deeper. I recently attended a meeting on hospital finance that one participant ruefully described as the 28th on the topic before restating his organization's same position from the beginning.

In place of unwieldy stakeholder committees, government agencies should convene smaller advisory committees with a specific charge and timeline. Such committees should hold public meetings and take public comment. The committees can ask those with special expertise, unique experiences, and even financial interest to provide input not only on the problem but also on creative solutions. Moreover, these committees can respond thoughtfully to all perspectives raised before making clearly understood recommendations that serve the common good.

This is hardly a new idea. For example, in October 1927, the Committee to Study and Report on Advisory Committees for Official Public Health Nursing presented its findings at the American Public Health Association meeting in Cincinnati, Ohio. The committee noted that the best advice comes from individuals who "serve without pay" and "represent no partisan politics nor self-seeking interests in the community" and who should "be chosen for their intelligence, public spirit, generally known integrity and good will."[4]

Recently, the state of Rhode Island asked a small group of experts to engage in extensive public consultation on the challenge of addiction and to make a set of strategic recommendations. At an early public meeting, Dr. Josiah Rich of Brown Alpert Medical School announced, "Our goal here is not to make everybody in this room happy. Our goal is to cut down on overdose deaths."[5]

With regard to the many stakeholder sessions already being planned for 2017, it's not too late to break out the dictionary and use more specific and helpful terms. Agencies should also consider whether a neutral expert committee should be added to the policymaking mix. One can only hope that within a year or two, we all might be working together on banishing other phrases listed by Lake Superior State University from the health policy lexicon, including "community of learners," "factoid," and "kick the can down the road."

References

1. Lake Superior State University. Lake Superior State University's 41st annual list of banished words. January 1, 2016. http://www.lssu.edu/banished/. Accessed June 13, 2016.
2. Centers for Disease Control and Prevention. Introduction to program evaluation for public health programs: a self-study guide. May 11, 2012. http://www.cdc.gov/eval/guide/step1/. Accessed June 13, 2016.
3. *Oxford English Dictionary*, 3rd Edition, 2004.
4. Committee to Study and Report on Advisory Committees for Official Public Health Nursing. Advisory committees for official public health nursing. *Am J Public Health (NY)*. 1927;17(12):1235–1239.
5. Bogdan J. RI's newly created drug-addiction and overdose task force holds first meeting. Providence Journal. August 19, 2015. http://www.providencejournal.com/article/20150819/NEWS/150819286. Accessed June 13, 2016.

APPENDIX 4 | Flint, Michigan, and the Failure of Public Agencies

REPRINTED FROM *The Journal of the American Medical Association* courtesy of the American Medical Association.

On my first day as health commissioner in Baltimore in December 2005, the chief counsel to the city gave me some advice: When you see a problem, fix it. Don't let your first instinct be to wonder who caused the problem, or to wait for every possible detail, or to defer to others. He said that the most important question the public will ever have about any problem is whether it has been fixed. And then he added, in an unwavering, deep voice, that fixing the problem is the right thing to do.

After the disastrous decisions that led to contamination of the water supply in Flint, Michigan, public agencies stumbled again by failing to identify the problem and respond quickly. Delays led to brutal assessments of governmental inaction and likely played a role in the resignation of senior state and federal officials. It took the courageous work of a professor and a pediatrician to force public leaders to pay attention to a health crisis.

Whenever government agencies founder, some find fault in their leaders for heartlessness, ignorance, or incompetence (or a combination of all three). Yet there are also reasons why even well-intentioned and otherwise effective government officials may fail to recognize and fix problems. Without excusing any of the failures in Flint, it is worth considering whether these factors may have played a role there.

The blind spot for crisis. It is no secret that public officials, just like everyone else, prefer good news to bad news. A tap of the keyboard sends happy news releases and upbeat emails to the public, the media, and elected representatives. Agencies use positive news to generate internal pride and external momentum.

The emphasis on good news makes it more difficult to acknowledge bad news. Problems require more than words; they require attention, and many underfunded offices are stretched thin just meeting their daily obligations. Responding to a health or environmental challenge means intense focus, rapid decisionmaking, and robust engagement with communities; practically speaking, releasing bad news can require pulling staff from other important activities for days if not weeks or months. As a result, officials are susceptible to wishful thinking that concerns will resolve by themselves. In the case of Flint, some public officials apparently spent time developing reassuring press statements rather than planning a comprehensive response.

The organizational chart trap. Although public agencies can be quite large, any given technical topic is likely to be understood by only a few staff members located in a corner of the organizational chart. This is the group responsible for setting policy on the topic; it is also the group most likely to field questions about concerns that may arise.

If a crisis is brewing in an area of specialized knowledge, such as whether water from a new supply source has received adequate treatment, agency leaders need to assess the facts quickly and effectively. Relying on the same people responsible for having made key decisions in the first place risks falling into a trap of false reassurance. A better approach is to seek outside expert input. This apparently did not happen in Flint until it was too late.

Legal quicksand. When an agency leader is considering a bold course of action to address an unexpected problem, at least one person inside an agency is likely to ask, "Are we allowed to do that?" Legal concerns may be entirely appropriate. What often happens, however, is that leaders hold off on all action, including permissible steps, until the questions are resolved. As some involved in the Flint crisis have now discovered, an extended delay for legal review is impossible to justify after the crisis becomes widely known.

A better approach is for public officials to talk promptly and candidly about the crisis, explaining what options are under consideration. A clear statement setting out the facts about a public health hazard may even lead to voluntary action without the need for the agency to exercise legal authority.

Missing warning signs. Many problems come to light as a result of external investigations—from journalists, auditors, inspectors general, and others. Nearly always, the agency has a chance to spot clues about what is happening during the investigation and move fast to limit the damage. For example, a reporter may confront a health agency with uncomfortable facts or an auditor may ask for an unusual set of records. These are precious opportunities for public officials to recognize whether there is, in fact, a major crisis brewing and respond. Yet few agencies are set up to review these warning signs fairly and systematically and figure out if something is truly awry.

Failing to take advantage of early signals of trouble should be called "GSA moments," after the epic failure five years ago of the General Services Administration (GSA) to promptly recognize and address management failures that led to lavish parties held at the public's expense. By the time the Office of the Inspector General released its report, it was too late for the agency. In the case of Flint, concerns expressed by citizens, journalists, and outside scientists provided multiple opportunities for public officials to dig further into the problem, but they led to GSA moments instead.

The responsibility conundrum. An agency taking responsibility for fixing a problem can find itself blamed for having caused it in the first place. Why? The public will assume that the agency is acting to address the consequences of its own making. Countering this assumption can be difficult—and counterproductive. Moving forward to get a job done is often incompatible with casting blame on others, especially those whose assistance is needed in a collaborative effort. Success may require giving others a pass (as well as, perhaps, an opportunity at redemption).

Yet a common phobia among public officials is the fear of being held accountable for a problem for which others share responsibility. This is not difficult to understand in a world of judgmental journalists, partisan political conflict, and social media. However, when multiple agencies are circling around the same crisis, as in Flint, this phobia can lead to paralysis, without any agency stepping forward and embracing the challenge.

Effective public agencies are able to surmount all of these obstacles. Their leaders keep an eye out for the lurking crisis; they look outside for expert assistance when appropriate; they do not permit legal considerations to sap urgency; they react quickly to warning signs; and they embrace responsibility.

They do so not because they are sure to be rewarded for their actions at the end of the day, because there is no such assurance in public service. They do so because it's the right thing to do.

APPENDIX 5 | On Fear, Distrust, and Ebola

REPRINTED FROM *The Journal of the American Medical Association* courtesy of the American Medical Association.

Soon after the first US case of Ebola was diagnosed in Dallas, I decided that Maryland's Department of Health and Mental Hygiene should have a press conference (http://bit.ly/1Ajy09F). With leading infectious disease experts from the University of Maryland and Johns Hopkins, we answered questions from virtually every news outlet in the area for about 45 minutes.

After the health care workers became infected in Dallas, we called the media back for another press conference(http://bit.ly/14EqDAu). It involved the same team, plus Maryland's governor, Martin O'Malley. Later, after we designated 3 facilities to care for patients with Ebola should federally funded beds not be available, we did it yet again, adding experts from the MedStar Health System, a nonprofit, community-based health system that serves the Baltimore/Washington region (http://1.usa.gov/158073d).

Effective communication during a public health emergency requires a carefully orchestrated effort. When it's my job to be the conductor, my goal is not only for the team to play the right notes, but also to make sure that listeners can hear the melody.

During the 3 press conferences, our notes were the details: how the Ebola virus is transmitted, how personal protective equipment is worn, and how the state's emergency medical services and hospital system will respond if there is a suspect case.

But the real value of public health communications, especially during emergencies, is the melody, the underlying message. Our simple melody was that the state and the leading health care institutions in Maryland are present, focused, and working together to protect the public.

Fear during epidemics is based in distrust. People are quick to doubt experts, they criticize health officials for any perceived mistake, and they wonder aloud why more attention is not being paid to worst-case scenarios. As one frightened Texas congressman memorably said, "Every outbreak novel or zombie movie you see starts with somebody from the government sitting in front of a panel like this saying there's nothing to worry about (http://bit.ly/1FqnQd5)."

The distrust extends beyond the health care system. People question whether employers are doing enough to protect the workplace and whether schools are doing enough to protect children. They look sideways at the person next to them on the subway, or on the bus, or living next door.

Distrust unsettles and contributes to fear. Fear can lead to panic, as well as to discrimination, scapegoating, and even violence.

In an emergency, public officials who simply reflect public anxiety, distrust, and fear are not helping anyone. However, those who tell people not to be afraid may only wind up increasing the public's anxiety. A more promising approach is for government officials to join with respected health care leaders and organizations and address the public. Doing so demonstrates to the public that familiar and trusted sources of care are not going to abandon them. The family physician, in effect, is still on the job.

In late October, 3 governors announced a policy of quarantining all returning health care workers, suggesting that the public cannot even trust these heroes to stay out of harm's way(http://wapo.st/1G2ewyB). Maryland's governor, well experienced in emergency management, did not reflexively follow them. With his support, Maryland's Health Department stepped forward with a different approach, based on science and developed with our health care leaders and organizations. Our strategy distinguished between health care workers with known exposures and those without, and involved quarantine only as a last resort.

Thanks in part to the public health communications that preceded it, our message was broadly accepted(http://bsun.md/1AjB1a3). For the moment, at least, the public and media in Maryland were singing our song.

APPENDIX **6** | Of Mouse and Measles

REPRINTED FROM *The Journal of the American Medical Association* courtesy of the American Medical Association.

"Mickey Mouse Gets the Measles," reported one website. "Space Mountain with a Side of Measles," proclaimed a news blog, which could not resist adding that Measles was "not the name of an eighth 'Snow White' dwarf."

That a major measles outbreak began at the home of beloved cartoon characters is certainly attention-grabbing news. Most of the reporting and commentary, in turn, has focused on the role of declining vaccination rates. This concern is especially acute in specific communities, including Orange County, California, where the theme park is located, and where some private schools have immunization rates as low as 60%. A recent Kaiser study in *Pediatrics* found clusters of underimmunization in 5 areas of northern California.

Beyond the setting, there has not been much discussion of the significance of Disneyland to the story. "Don't expect a 'Disneyland effect' " improving immunization rates, wrote one health economist. Parental attitudes on vaccines are too fixed, and our attention spans too short, she wrote, to think that anything will change.

I disagree. My intuition is in line with that of some practicing pediatricians: Mickey, Minnie, Goofy, and friends can help change the terms of the discussion on vaccines.

The traditional framing of a vaccine controversy sets the evidence and judgment of scientists and clinicians against the skepticism of a small minority about the risks and benefits of specific immunizations. The playing field is science, and points are won with data.

On one side are the vast majority of pediatricians, myself included, who fully support the recommended vaccine schedule. Our perspective on the evidence indicates that the benefits of vaccines to children in our practices and to all children are far greater than the risks. (I was the dad who ran out to purchase pneumococcal vaccination with my own money during the narrow window after US Food and Drug Administration approval but before the recommendation for universal vaccination was implemented.)

On the other side are increasing numbers of parents who are concluding that the risk of vaccination to their children is greater than the potential benefit. They are willing to take the risk of illness and skip vaccination. As one California pediatrician close to many parents who refuse vaccination stated on his Facebook page, "Most anti-vaxers do believe vaccines work. They aren't willing to risk the side effects."

Pediatricians tend to respond to vaccine resistance by flooding parents with evidence of vaccine effectiveness and safety. The problem is that while information is important, overdoing it may backfire.

A recent Michigan study found that presenting facts to vaccine-refusing parents may actually have the effect of making them more reluctant to vaccinate. As Julie-Anne Leask, PhD, MPH, of the University of Sydney's School of Public Health in Australia, has written, "there is little empirical support for the hope that decision making about vaccination is based on 'facts' alone." She also warns clinicians to be careful of deluging parents with information that have the "opposite effect of polarising people into existing positions where . . . those opposed become more entrenched . . .." Her recommendation is for a more deliberate approach, reinforced by trusted leaders in a community, which emphasizes the benefits of "protecting children from threatening diseases."

And what better way to convey those benefits than to imagine a Disneyland where children and parents do not have to fear measles?

After many years of decline, measles is back, and outbreaks are just one sign of trouble. School systems are sending children who are not vaccinated home for weeks at a time. Parents of children with cancer and other conditions that preclude vaccination are becoming increasingly angry about the risk that nonvaccinating parents are causing.

As measles continues to spread, these skirmishes can be expected to extend past schools. It is reasonable to ask whether children with cancer and other underlying disorders should risk their health at Disneyland, at the movies, and in sports stadiums simply because other parents have rejected vaccination. Should a child in such a situation become seriously injured or die, pressure will grow for political leaders to protect the most vulnerable—and businesses will react to avoid liability. The Internet headline might one day read: No MMR, No Mickey Mouse.

"What . . . do non-vaxers want?" asked the California pediatrician close to many parents hesitant to accept pediatric recommendations. "They don't want to be discriminated against. They want to be able to attend school if they want (if not sick, of course). . . . They don't want it to even be an issue that affects social and family life."

Carefully and clearly, clinicians and community leaders together can respond to this sentiment: Not possible.

When it comes to life-threatening diseases, there is no having your cake and eating it too. There is no refusing to vaccinate but getting to do everything else just the same. When parents reject recommended vaccines, then a community can impose restrictions to protect the lives and health of other children.

States already make this decision with respect to schools. In 30 states, with rare exceptions, state law requires parents to immunize their children or agree not to send them to school. Twenty states have decided otherwise and permit broader exception language for parents. There are signs pressure is already growing for these laws to be strengthened.

The Disneyland outbreak illustrates beautifully that more is at stake for children than rare adverse effects. That's because vaccines do more than protect from disease. They provide a zone of safety around our children everywhere they go. They protect all children in case of illness with cancer or other disorders. Vaccines allow families to live in communities that are safer, more livable, and more fun.

Where doctors have tried and failed, they should consider calling in some reinforcements. I understand Donald Duck is available for consults.

APPENDIX 7 | On Working for Henry Waxman

REPRINTED FROM *The Millbank Quarterly* courtesy of the Millbank Memorial Fund.

My first meeting with Congressman Henry A. Waxman, the giant of health policy who recently announced that he was retiring after 40 years in Congress, came soon after I started working on his staff. I had left a full-time medical career on an academic track to join the staff as a junior member and had moved with my family to Washington, DC.

I sat low on the couch in his office, facing him in a chair. "What do you want to accomplish in this position?" he asked. There was a long, awkward pause. Then I said, "I'd like to work on national health insurance." He grimaced. "You won't be long for this job," he said.

The year was 2001. President George W. Bush was in the White House, and Congress was under Republican control.

"I don't want you to spend your time pushing for something that is not going to happen anytime soon," Waxman added. "Let's find areas where we can make progress, and we'll wait for the right time for national health insurance."

What followed was, for me, a 4-year immersion course in health policy and politics. I had a front-row seat as Congressman Waxman accomplished more in the minority party than most members of Congress accomplish in their entire careers. He was a chef using only readily available ingredients but somehow was able to assemble one surprising dish after the other.

Congressman Waxman released evidence-based reports and letters with the same frequency that his colleagues put out press statements. With clear methods and exhaustive references, the reports brought data to bear on critical policy questions and, in the process, framed those questions in a way that pointed naturally to a solution.

For example, during my time on his staff, Congressman Waxman wrote the US Olympic Committee about the potential harm of new Taekwondo rules that encouraged children to knock out one another with blows to the head[1] (the policy was soon reversed)[2]; queried the US Food and Drug Administration (FDA) about the safety of nicotine lollipops[3] (which were quickly removed from the market)[4]; asked GlaxoSmithKline about its withdrawal of support for a critical international HIV trial[5] (Glaxo changed its mind the next day)[6]; detailed how the Bush administration had altered a report on health disparities[7] (the original version was later released)[8]; and wrote to food manufacturers about their erroneous nutritional claims for rice-based "milk" products[9] (leading to revised packaging for leading brands).

Because Congressman Waxman encouraged his staff to connect the dots between discrete issues, we were able to put together a comprehensive report on the Bush administration's misuse of science,[10] helping define its shortcomings on a range of issues for the media and the public, as well as providing a language for resisting new threats to science-based policy.

While his criticism of the Republican administration made the most headlines, Congressman Waxman also was generous with support when called for. He once wrote critically of errors in a report on preventable causes of death coauthored by the director of the Centers for Disease Control and Prevention. But when those errors were addressed in a letter to the editor, he thanked her publicly and considered the matter closed. He supported the Bush administration's position on vaccine safety because it was the correct one, despite criticism from the Republican leaders of his committee. His integrity was one of the most important reasons why Congressman Waxman's reputation and influence grew throughout his tenure in Congress.

It also made working for him a great pleasure. From time to time, a left-leaning interest group would come to me asking that Congressman Waxman sign a letter or support a position that was not terribly well thought out. I would do my best to decline, politely. Nonetheless, I recall managing to infuriate one caller, who pointedly asked me whether the good congressman was aware that a "right-winger" was secretly working on his staff. She then demanded to talk with Congressman Waxman personally. I replied: "I'm happy to ask the congressman to speak to you, but first let's think about how that conversation is going to go. You will ask him to sign your letter, and I'll point out errors that are unnecessary and will ultimately be used to attack him. He won't sign the letter, and your credibility with him will be gone forever." My caller chose instead to revise the letter.

Congressman Waxman was the driving force and lead sponsor behind numerous legislative advances in health policy, including multiple insurance expansions in the Medicaid program, the Ryan White Care Act for HIV/AIDS, the Family Smoking Prevention and Tobacco Control Act, the Vaccine Injury Compensation Program, and the Hatch-Waxman Act, which created the market for generic drugs.

What do these topics have in common? Only that there was a need and an opportunity to pass legislation to advance the health of the nation. Rather than expend all his energy on proposals that had no chance of passage, Congressman Waxman found opportunities in the crises of the moment. He spoke out with tremendous moral force, and he also worked behind the scenes when such an approach was more effective.

Under his signature, our committee staff conducted a survey of every juvenile detention center in the nation and found that more than half were holding children unnecessarily because community services were not available. Then when it came time to release the report, we did so with a Republican senator in order to maximize our reach and impact.[11]

I brought to Congressman Waxman the problem of the FDA's deregulating the sale of nonprescription contact lenses, under a new legal theory holding that such lenses were technically not medical devices. Children were purchasing these lenses over the counter, developing severe corneal injuries or infections, and risking blindness. He found a Republican member of Congress to work with, and we quietly moved legislation through both the House and the Senate to become Public Law 109–96. Few took notice of his guiding hand.

A critical question in policy and politics is whether a particular compromise is a good deal, or in the language of political science professors, is half a loaf of bread better than none?

If there were a final exam for my immersion course working for Congressman Waxman, this would be the only question. And after watching his pragmatic approach yield results time and again, my answer would be yes—but only when the half a loaf creates the conditions that can lead to further progress later. Congressman Waxman always had an eye on the next step, the one that would include more people, extend lifesaving benefits even further, or have a greater lasting impact.

The Affordable Care Act—our nation's closest answer to national health insurance—is one such compromise. The president and Congress, with the leadership of Congressman Waxman, took advantage of an unusual opportunity to extend health coverage to tens of millions of Americans and reform our nation's delivery system. While the law is far from perfect, its implementation is creating new expectations for the availability and affordability of health insurance, the role of prevention, and the need for value in health care services.

Such expectations will help shape the steps forward for our health care system. This time, however, Congressman Waxman will not be in Congress to lead the effort. This is the nation's loss and a challenge to the rest of us to honor his legacy.

References

1. Letter from Rep. Henry A. Waxman and Rep. Jesse Jackson Jr. to William C. Martin, Acting President, US Olympic Committee. April 24, 2004. http://oversight-archive.waxman.house.gov/documents/20040628070626--12542.pdf Accessed March 5, 2014.
2. Officials worry about athlete head trauma. Associated Press. May 20, 2004.
3. Letter from Rep. Henry A. Waxman to Secretary of the US Dept of Health and Human Services Tommy Thompson. April 3, 2002. http://oversight-archive.waxman.house.gov/documents/20040827160232--53520.pdf Accessed March 5, 2014.
4. FDA melts nicotine lollipops. CNN. April 10, 2002. http://money.cnn.com/2002/04/10/news/fda_lollipops/index.htm. Accessed April 28, 2014.
5. Waxman Henry A, Garnier JP. Letter from Rep. Glaxo Pharmaceuticals. June 30, 2004. http://oversight-archive.waxman.house.gov/documents/20040817123439--66837.pdf Accessed March 5, 2014.
6. Glaxo to remain part of HIV trial in poor countries. Wall Street Journal. July 1, 2004.
7. A case study in politics and science: changes to the National Healthcare Disparities Report. Report of the minority staff of the Government Reform Committee. January 2004. http://oversight-archive.waxman.house.gov/documents/20040901170729--77795.pdf Accessed March 5, 2014.
8. Bloche MG. Health care disparities—science, politics, and race. N Engl J Med. 2004; 350(15):1568–1570. [PubMed]
9. Letter from Rep. Henry A. Waxman to FDA Commissioner Andrew C. von Eschenbach. November 17, 2005. http://oversight-archive.waxman.house.gov/documents/20051117130206—26259.pdf Accessed March 5, 2014.